Medical Escort & Repatriation Course, International

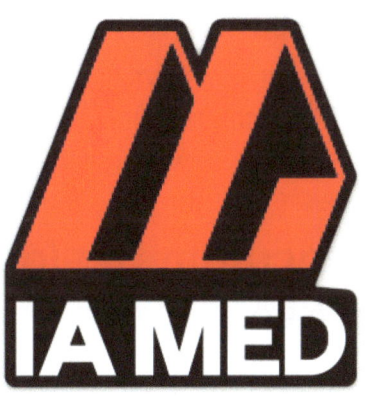

Jessica Peltz, BSN, RN, CFRN, EMT-P

Chris Smetana, AS, NRP, FP-C, CCP-C

Lindsay Mauldin, RN, NRP, CFRN, FP-C, CCP-C

Jim Green, DC, NRP, FP-C

Editor
Francine King, MS, BA

Education Committee
Director: Lindsay V. Mauldin, RN, CFRN, CEN, NRP, FP-C, CCP-C
Lead Registered Nurse: Jacob A. Miller, MS, APRN, FNP-BC, AGACNP-BC, ACCNS-AG, CCRN, CFRN, NRP, FP-C
Lead Paramedic: Andy Fidino, NRP, FP-C

Medical Director
Mike Hudson, MD, EM, EMS
Air Medical Program Chief Medical Director
Level 1 ED Trauma Physician

Curriculum Designer
Jonathan Reed, BA, NRP, ATP, TP-C, FP-C, 18D

Cover/Graphic Designer
Mike Boone, BSN, RN, CFRN, CCRN

Reviewers
Jessica Horowitz, MS, BS, NRP, CCT-P
Brock Jenkins, FP-C, NRP
Jeremy Singleton, RN, CEN

Contributors
Stephen Avise, EMT-P
Liron Beltzer, M.D.
Walter Kerr, MS, NR-EMT-P, FP-C, CMTE
Hi Flying Air Ambulance

DISCLAIMER

All rights reserved. No part of the material protected by this copyright may be reproduced or utilized in any form, electronic or mechanical, including photocopying, recording, or by any information storage and retrieval system, without written permission from the authors & the copyright owner.

The content, statements, views, and opinions herein are the sole expression of the respective authors and Immediate Action Medicine, INC.

The procedures and protocols in this book are based on the most current recommendations of responsible medical sources at the time of publication. Immediate Action Medicine, INC makes no guarantee as to and assumes no responsibility for, the correctness, sufficiency, or completeness of such information or recommendations. Other or additional safety measures may be required under particular circumstances.

This textbook is intended solely as a study guide to the appropriate procedures to be employed when rendering care as part of a medical escort or repatriation. It is not intended as a standard of care required in an emergency, because circumstances and the patient's physical condition can widely vary from one situation to another. It is not intended that this study guide shall, in any way, advise emergency personnel concerning legal authority to perform the activities or procedures discussed. Such local determination should be made only with the aid of legal counsel, your medical director, and your agency's protocols.

MERCI: Medical Escort & Repatriation Course, International is an independent publication. It has not been authorized, sponsored, or otherwise approved by the owners of the trademarks or service marks referenced in this product.

Reference herein to any specific commercial product, process, or service by trade name, trademark, manufacturer, or otherwise does not constitute or imply its endorsement or recommendation by Immediate Action Medicine, INC, and such reference shall not be used for IA MED ©2020 *MERCI: Medical Escort & Repatriation Course, International* study guide in advertising or product endorsement purposes. All trademarks displayed are the trademarks of the parties noted herein.

There may be images in this book that feature models; these models do not necessarily endorse, represent, or participate in the activities represented in the images. Any screenshots in this product are for educational and instructive purposes only. Any individuals and scenarios featured in the case studies or examples throughout this study guide may be real or fictitious but are used for instructional purposes only.

Copyright

Copyright © 2020 by Immediate Action Medicine, INC

All Rights Reserved

ISBN

9798554907821

Printed in the United States of America

DEDICATION

Medical Escort & Repatriation Course, International is dedicated to all of the physicians, registered nurses, paramedics, and respiratory therapists that were put into difficult travel and logistical situations without any prior training. It is dedicated to those that had to "figure it out on their own" and just make it happen.

There are a million shades of grey while conducting commercial escorts and repatriations. Much of what we do every day stems from frequent encouragement and bolstering to our patients- helping them realize that they CAN get home commercially despite how tiring and complex it can be. We, the clinicians, have the easy part. Our ill and injured patients are the ones working hard to make their repatriation possible.

This course is also dedicated to all of the medical escort programs that struggle with staff orientation, training and compliance. With the lack of unified medical escort education; it is our intention to make this a solution for you as well. You will know that what is required of accreditation compliance is provided in a singular location.

It is our goal that this is merely the first step in medical escort clinician education. With your continued input, this course will grow and evolve to meet the ever-changing needs of the industry. Please share your experiences and feedback with us at support@iamed.us

ACKNOWLEDGEMENTS

First, I would like to thank Chris, Zack and Lindsay for being open-hearted when I became a part of the team. While I see myself more as an administrator than an instructor, I truly felt that this topic needed some solidarity and relevancy. The entire IA MED team has been so eager to see this course come to fruition, and for that I am humbled.

I also want to thank YOU. YOU are the reason for the Medical Escort & Repatriation Course, International. Without the struggles of learning as you go, or having to "figure it out," the inspiration behind this course would be non-existent.

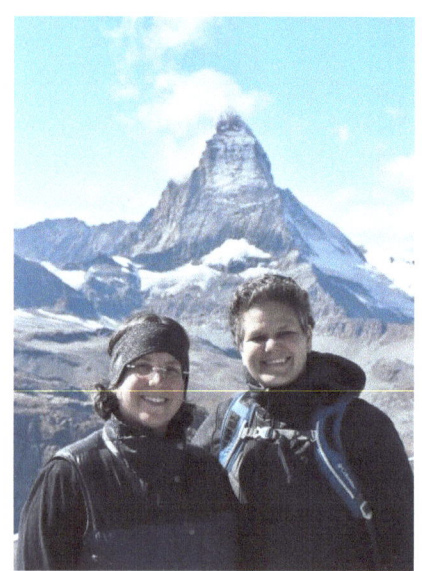

Lastly, but most certainly not least, I would like to thank my wife, Amanda. Without her dedication and support, this idea that I have had in my mind for years never would have become something tangible and practical for others to learn, enjoy and share.

Countless hours of a shared office, conflicting video calls and the occasional dislike in music selections.

She is by far the most patient and understanding person I know.

-Jessica

I personally would like to thank the IA MED Team for their hard work and selfless dedication to help IA MED grow. Their contributions to the company and the impact they have left on both their students and the industry has been immeasurable. It truly takes a TEAM to make this happen and am thankful for our IA MED Family!

To my friend and business partner Jon Reed, thank you for your support, mentorship, and all the heavy lifting and sacrifices you and Kate have had to endure to help make IA MED an industry leader. Thank you, brother. "Ride or Die"

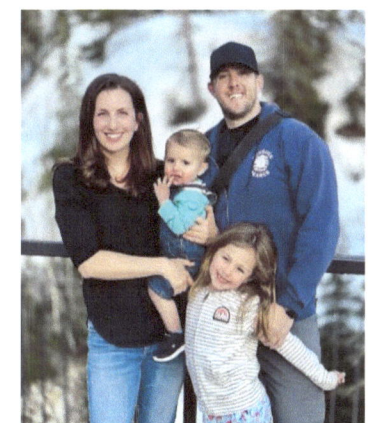

To my friends and family, I can never repay the debt for all the sacrifices you have had to endure to make this book and IA MED possible.

To my daughter, Shay, thank you for always showing me the love and fun in life. You are a beautiful soul. To my son, Ben, thank you for being my sidekick watching Fireman Sam with me while working late.

Lastly, to my wife Susie, I know how hard you have struggled with my long hours, no days off, and me continually being away while growing IA MED. You have a given part of yourself to help me aspire to achieve my dreams. I can never repay that debt, but I always promise to be the loving husband by your side and give you all of me while trying every day. I am thankful to have been your partner and on this crazy adventure for the past 20 years. I truly thank you for your sacrifices and love your face!

-Chris

This book would not have been possible without the support and encouragement of those in our industry and the desire for better education. Jon and Chris, thank you for the opportunity to be part of the IA Med family. It has truly been a fun ride, I'm lucky to have such great partners, and I look forward to where we go next.

To my mentors in the industry, thank you for always pushing me, encouraging me, and motivating me to spread my wings. I am so lucky to have such an array of people to bounce ideas off of, all over the globe.

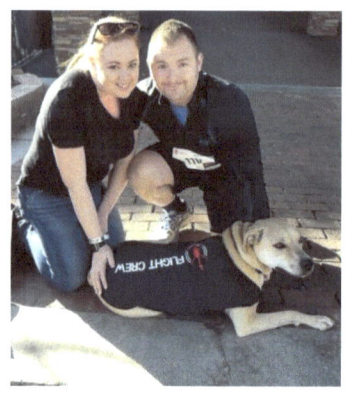

To my mom, thank you for always believing in me, especially on the days I didn't believe in myself. You have supported me in ways I can't begin to count, even when my path has been the one less traveled.

To my husband Chuck, you're my bar. You have given endless support to help me achieve where I am today and continue to push me to be a better version of myself. You have been patient when I'm cranky from trying to fit 50 hours of work into a 24-hour day, or when I'm exhausted from traveling too much. Words cannot express how fortunate I feel to have both you and Pickles by my side through thick and thin. Thank you for your sacrifice and everything you do.

-Lindsay

PREFACE

Immediate Action Medicine, Inc. ("IA MED") is a disabled veteran-owned small business that provides cutting-edge specialty medical training, ranging from aeromedical critical care to austere tactical medicine. Our proprietary system has been continuously developed and refined since 2011, using a comprehensive data-driven approach.

MERCI: Medical Escort & Repatriation Course, International is an addition to the IA MED education platform to take aeromedical and critical care in commercial transport to the next level of patient care and management.

Since 2011, IA MED® has helped thousands of students launch careers as advanced prehospital and critical care professionals by providing the most comprehensive, flexible, and accessible critical care education in the nation. By presenting complex medical concepts through straightforward instruction, we make learning critical care simple - regardless of your current medical ability or experience.

Our unique approach to advanced medical education has made IA MED® the industry-standard and a fan-favorite among paramedics, nurses, and other industry providers.

MERCI: Medical Escort & Repatriation Course, International will review the essential information needed to successfully complete a medical escort or repatriation mission. This includes administrative, logistical and clinical information.

The information learned here is intended to supplement your program's specific training, medical protocols and policies & procedures. Some sections will provide you with QR codes to visit specific websites or to watch brief, supplemental videos. Modern phones have built in QR readers into the camera. If your phone does not, we highly encourage you to download a free QR reader app for a better experience.

Throughout the manual, you will see the following icon:
It is meant to make you aware of a pearl of wisdom gathered from industry experts in the field. These small bits of information can make-or-break your success while conducting commercial repatriations.

This is EMS. Re-imagined.

TABLE OF CONTENTS

DISCLAIMER I

DEDICATION III

ACKNOWLEDGEMENTS IV

PREFACE VII

TABLE OF CONTENTS VIII

MEDICAL ESCORT GENERAL INFORMATION 2
- What is a Medical Escort? 2
- Roles Within Your Program 3
- HIPAA, GDPR and Patient Privacy 3
- Quality Management 4
- Compliance 4
- Medical Escort Policies & Procedures 5
- Medical Protocols 5
- Client Relations 5
- Medical Clearance and Fitness-To-Fly 5
- Customer Service 6
- Conclusion 7

COMMERCIAL AIRLINE HEALTH & WELLBEING 8
- Just Culture 8
- Communications Strategies 8
- General Travel Advice & Suggestions 9
- Aircraft, Tarmac & Emergency Safety 9
- Personal Health & Wellbeing 14
- Infection Control 19
- Infectious Diseases 20
- Conclusion 24

COMMERCIAL TRANSPORT ENVIRONMENT 25
- Mission Planning & Following 25
- Ground Transport Operations 26
- Flight Physiology & Stressors of Transport 28
- Medical Equipment, Oxygen, Classes Of Travel & Stretchers 34
- In-Flight Management 36
- Putting it all Together 40
- Conclusion 42

CLINICAL GUIDELINES AND EMERGENCIES 43

Disaster & Triage 43
Activating a Medical Emergency Onboard 44
Anatomy & Physiology – 'Special Populations' 45
Pediatric Emergencies 48
Adult Emergencies 49
    Neurological & Neurosurgical Emergencies 49
    Psychiatric Emergencies 55
    Respiratory Emergencies 56
    Basic Airway Management 59
    Cardiac Emergencies 61
    Gastrointestinal Disorders 63
    Metabolic & Endocrine Disorders 65
    Pituitary Disorders 66
    Environmental & Toxicology Emergencies 67
    Trauma Patient Management 71
Miscellaneous Basic Pharmacology 76
Conclusion 77

ALS & CRITICAL CARE IN THE COMMERCIAL ENVIRONMENT 78

Equipment 78
Critical Care Concepts 79
    Neuro Patients 79
    Respiratory Patients 81
    Advanced Airway Management 82
    Airway Assessment 82
    Equipment & Patient Positioning 84
    Rapid Sequence Intubation (RSI) & Pharmacology 86
    Ventilator Patient Management 92
    Ventilator Settings & Modes 94
    Cardiac Patients 100
Conclusion 103

QUICK REFERENCE CHARTS 104

MERCI TRAVEL CHECKLIST 109

REVIEW QUESTIONS 110

REFERENCES 129

x

MEDICAL ESCORT & REPATRIATION COURSE, INTERNATIONAL

We recognized that there is a lack in unified and relevant Medical Escort & Repatriation education available to the many medical professionals involved in this industry.

If you are currently involved in or wish to be involved in the commercial air transfer of individuals requiring medical monitoring, this is for you!

This course has been designed for the veteran provider, as well as clinicians new to commercial repatriations.

While we did our very best to include all possible aspects of the industry, your experience may vary from what we discuss.

Please note: policies, procedures, treatment modalities and medications may vary from your program's scope of practice. The topics discussed are done so in a *general* way. Please, always refer to your program's documentation. Some topics discussed are required for programs seeking or maintaining industry accreditation.

The terms "medical escort" and "repatriation" will be used interchangeably throughout this manual, as well as "clinician" and "medical escort."

If you have an experience to share that will improve the curriculum, please contact: support@iamed.us.

Course Objectives

1. Identify a clinically appropriate patient for commercial transport
2. Describe the safety implications of commercial air travel, including clinician responsibility in crew resource management and personal health and wellbeing
3. Explain the challenges that surround the commercial transport environment
4. Apply flight physiology to clinical patient conditions as part of human factors and forward thinking

MEDICAL ESCORT GENERAL INFORMATION

What is a Medical Escort?

Medical escorts are patient transports that occur on commercial airlines. They are often seen as a financially reasonable alternative to air ambulance. These patients can require routine, or basic; care while others may require a higher level of care like advanced life support (ALS) or critical care stretchers (CC).

The routine, or basic medical escort patients typically do not require a higher level of care and are easily deemed fit-to-fly (FTF) commercially. Many medical escort patients were on holiday and became ill or injured. Some may seek treatment at specialized medical centers.

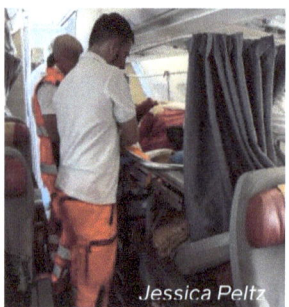

The ALS medical escort patient may require additional clearance or screening by the airline. These patients may require basic cardiac monitoring and IV medication administration which can be done in the business/first class cabin or via stretcher.

CC escort patients may require the use of a stretcher. These transfers can require 3-7 days to arrange with the airline, including medical clearance.

Not every patient is appropriate for commercial repatriation. This is determined by a thorough review process by your program's clinical supervisors, airline medical desk personnel, the overseeing physician and insurance company case managers (if applicable). Fit-to-fly must be provided by the treating physician and approved by the airline.

When possible, prior to departing to the patient's location, obtain an updated medical report to confirm the patient's suitability for commercial travel. This allows you to critically analyze the most up-to-date information to confirm the patient's suitability for commercial travel.

Roles Within Your Program

- Medical Director
    - Legally responsible for the care provided
    - Defines scope of practice
    - Approves medical/treatment protocols, either on- or off-line
- Program Manager
    - Heavily involved in the growth and development of the program.
- Clinical Supervisor
    - Responsible for the day-to-day clinical operations

Depending on the size of your program, one person may be responsible for more than one role. For example, the Program Manager and Clinical Supervisor may be the same person— and that person may also be the Quality Manager.

HIPAA, GDPR and Patient Privacy

HIPAA is the Health Insurance Portability and Accountability Act. Enacted in 1996 by U.S. Congress, according to the California Department of Health Care Services, it "requires the protection and confidential handling of protected health information."

GDPR is the General Data Protection Regulation. It is an EU (European Union) law addressing data protection and privacy. (gdpr-info.eu)

Your program may have its own patient privacy regulations, including those that follow national guidelines. As a general rule, you should follow the "minimum necessary" rule when discussing protected health information, or PHI.

Be aware that the captain of the commercial aircraft is permitted to know medical/clinical data on the patient.

Protected Health Information is defined as:
- Past, present or future physical or mental health of an individual
- Provision of health care to an individual
- Past, present or future payment for the provision of health care **together with any of the identifiers below**:
    - Name, social security number, geographic subdivisions smaller than a state, all elements of dates (except year) like birth, admissions, etc., telephone numbers, full face photographic images, etc. (1)

Essentially, any routine privacy rules you follow as a medical provider must still be followed and maintained while conducting a medical escort.

For electronic devices, today's standard is a password lock/screen. Depending on your national regulations and your program's policies, additional security may be required when storing medical records electronically. **Remember**: do not leave any device open/unlocked with private data visible. Paper records can be easily displaced. **Keep all paper records together, in a folder or envelope in your patient's carry-on bag**.

Quality Management

Your program has its own internal quality management program. Some items that are monitored include:
- Patient Care
- Safety incidents with metrics
- Medical equipment maintenance and failures/errors
- Utilization review (appropriate mode of transport [air/ground], appropriately credentialed clinician, appropriate class of travel, etc.)
- Customer satisfaction
- Team member satisfaction

The Quality Manager is responsible for identifying issues involved in transport, mitigating them and monitoring future occurrences. A lot of this information is reported directly by you!

Compliance

Every medical transport program must adhere to local, national and international rules, regulations and laws.

In the U.S., this includes EMTALA, Office of Inspector General, anti-kickback laws, etc.

EMTALA is the Emergency Medical Treatment and Labor Act. It is a U.S. federal law that requires any individual presenting to an emergency room to be evaluated and treated/stabilized within the abilities of the facility, regardless of ability to pay. It was designed to prevent the transfer of uninsured patients to a different hospital. (acep.org)

Internationally, these laws may vary, and you should refer to your manager.

Some programs may be required to carry the following insurance:
- Worker's Compensation
  - Cover's medical expenses of a worker that becomes ill or injured as a result of performing job duties
- Medical Malpractice
- Clinician Travel Insurance

Medical Escort Policies & Procedures

Your transport program has unique policies and procedures that have been developed, reviewed and approved by your leaders. For any questions or clarifications, refer to them.

Medical Protocols

Medical protocols are physician's orders that have been approved by your medical director for off-line (no direct communication available with your medical director) use.

For example and depending on your protocols, if your patient complains of a headache, you are permitted to medicate them with acetaminophen or ibuprofen without consulting with your medical director.

If communicating with your medical director *on-line* (telephone, SMS, email), he or she may authorize additional medication or interventions that you would otherwise not be permitted to provide. On-line authorizations are physician orders.

Client Relations

Medical escort trips are sourced from several avenues:
- Private pay
- An individual pays your company directly for services to move their loved one
- Other air medical transport providers
- Travel Insurance/Assistance

Subscribers to travel insurance notify their insurer that they are ill and require case management/involvement. Once the patient has been evaluated, treated and case reviewed, the travel insurance medical director will approve the commercial transfer and notify your company.

Medical Clearance and Fitness-To-Fly

Medical Clearance and FTF is completed by the treating physician. If working with travel insurance or travel assistance, the medical director will also provide a "fit-to-fly" and provide travel recommendations.

For private pay patients, your program will work with the treating physician to obtain medical clearance. Finally, your program must obtain medical clearance from the airline medical desk prior to the transport. This is accomplished by the completion and submission of a Medical Information Form, or MEDIF, for short.

Regardless, a MEDIF for each airline being utilized must be completed and signed by your medical director as part of the medical clearance process. A sample MEDIF is included.

It is vital to understand that FTF an air ambulance (AA) mission differs vastly from FTF for commercial repatriation. While there are few actual contraindications to fixed-wing AA transfers, the same cannot be said for commercial missions.

For example, your patient may be fully ambulatory and on a non-rebreather mask. This patient is NOT a commercial candidate and would be better served by an AA. Alternatively, while a fully ambulatory patient on 2 LPM nasal cannula *may* be transported by AA, this particular patient is appropriate for commercial transfer.

There are factors in deciding on air ambulance vs. commercial escort:
1. The patient's FTF status
2. Diagnosis
3. Clinical care required
4. Location
    a. It is not uncommon to do a "wing-to-wing" with an air ambulance as part of the commercial repatriation/escort.
        i. A "wing-to-wing" transfer is the transfer of a patient from one aircraft to another. Example: a patient arrives in Frankfurt (FRA) from a remote location (with limited commercial service) via air ambulance. The patient is then transferred to a commercial aircraft for flight to Los Angeles (LAX).
5. Timeline
    a. Air ambulance can be activated in hours for transport while commercial can take days for transport

Once fitness-to-fly is confirmed, the airline must review the information and provide medical clearance. Without medical clearance, you and your patient may not be permitted to board.

Customer Service

Customer service is invaluable in this industry. It is far more beneficial to be polite and courteous while traveling the world.

External clients include your patient, your company's client, insurance companies, ground transport providers, airport and airline personnel, to name a few.

Patient care - Don't forget that you are caring for one individual for what could be a lengthy amount of time. Customer service is 100% vital in this industry. This is an amazing opportunity to make a positive impact in someone's life during a very stressful time through the one-on-one care you provide.
When conducting a commercial transfer, there are a lot of factors that are out of your control. How you handle those unexpected occurrences will show your patient, the client and your program how well you function under stressful circumstances.

Conclusion

There are many moving parts to successfully conducting a commercial repatriation. Ensure your patient's privacy is observed and respected at all times and follow the "minimum necessary rule."

Your program has processes in place to ensure compliance, as well as your success. Refer to your company's materials.

Remember also that this industry centered on customer service – from your patient to the client to airline cabin crew!

COMMERCIAL AIRLINE HEALTH & WELLBEING 2

Just Culture

Just Culture is a way of thinking and operating that puts safety on the forefront, while acknowledging that there are barriers to the safe environment.

The principles include:
- Preoccupation with failure
    - *A problem is always there. Is it being reported? Are there barriers?*
- Reluctance to simplify
    - *That the failure is because of a systemic issue, not for a single, simple reason.*
- Sensitivity to operations
    - *Expected performance of operations can lead to a culture of "low expectation."*
- Deference to expertise
    - *Those that are involved in the 'incident' use their 'expertise' in the issue to provide learning opportunities*
- Resilience
    - *Errors happen- rather than being "disabled" by them, those involved recognize and intervene quickly and appropriately.*

If your program operates with a "Just Culture," it means that you are part of the solution!

Communications Strategies

Your communications department, clients and families all need to be kept up-to-date on the progress of the transport. Cellular phones with international coverage may be expected to be used. Your program will define requirements for keeping in touch while on a mission.

E-mail, texting and SMS are efficient ways to keep in touch, per your program's policies & procedures while maintaining patient privacy.

Many airlines offer WiFi, usually for purchase. Depending on your programs policies & procedures, you can access the onboard WiFi to ensure communication with your program and medical director, if needed.

General Travel Advice & Suggestions

Part of the allure of medical escorts is being able to travel and see the world. However, safety must remain in the forefront while traveling. When traveling, always observe your program's safety policies, which may address whether or not you are permitted to leave your hotel for reasons other than patient care related tasks.

Prior to departure, research local customs and traditions. Boring is best and it is not recommended to leave your hotel unless for mission specific tasks. If you do leave your hotel, stay in the "tourist" areas. The use of translation programs can make it easier for you to communicate while abroad.

Keep copies of your passport, licenses, certifications, immunizations, etc. in your mobile phone or packed in your bag. Monitor travel advisories and be familiar with the location of your home country's embassies and consulates.

Triple check for belongings, including those for the patient!

Don't forget to bring a power converter.. being out of the country with a dead cell phone can leave you feeling very isolated. Check the weather and pack accordingly.

Make yourself less of a target by minimizing jewelry, expensive luggage and clothing. Lastly, consider obtaining travel insurance in the event you become ill or injured yourself.

Aircraft, Tarmac & Emergency Safety

Airline Hazardous Materials

The rules for airline travel still apply to medical escorts. Be familiar with local, national and international regulations.

The Federal Aviation Administration provides an easy to use website:

PackSafe for Passengers

https://www.faa.gov/hazmat/packsafe/

Of importance: lithium batteries must be stored in carry-on bags due to the risk of fire.

Generally, as a passenger, you will not encounter any specific hazardous materials. However, it is important to understand what is and is not permitted on board. Lithium batteries are typically used in portable oxygen concentrators.

Commercial Aircraft Safety Considerations

Aviation safety is managed by the commercial airline itself. Your responsibilities include following the directives of the airline representatives on the ground and cabin crew for any safety briefings, procedures, etc. for both yourself AND your patient.

Security screenings will be conducted per local airport and national regulations. Assist with your patient 's luggage to ensure it meets the airline's regulations.

Pre-flight briefing elements include:
- Seat belt Operation (take-off and landing)
- Emergency Exit Operations
- Emergency Egress Procedure
- Cabin security requirements

Briefings are a legal and mandatory requirement. Take notice, turn off your portable electronic devices and LISTEN. You may have to explain them to your patient and will likely be assisting them if any emergencies occur.

If you are a medical escort with a patient, you will not be permitted to sit in the emergency exit rows – simply because of your patient will likely have limited mobility.

Safety on the Ramp or Tarmac

Safety around the commercial aircraft is vital. There may be times you will be moving about on an active ramp and there can be many hazards. Watch for cables and lines, moving vehicles, luggage, etc. It can also be very noisy so it is imperative you communicate clearly. Consider the use of hearing protection for yourself and patient.

Be mindful of:
- Jetway safety
- Stairs to the aircraft which may involve carrying the patient
- Use of ambu-lift for stretcher patients
- Walking from a bus to the airplane
- ALWAYS BE ALERT AND KEEP YOUR EYES OPEN

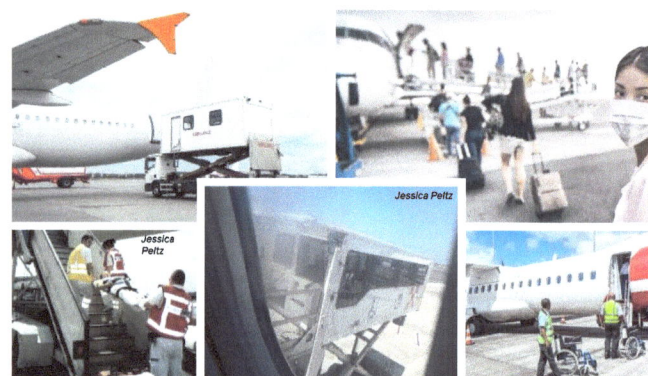

Inflight and Emergency Landing Procedures

In the event of an aircraft emergency, the cabin and cockpit crew will provide instructions to supplement the pre-flight safety briefing. Always apply your oxygen before helping others due to the time of useful consciousness.

There are many reasons for a commercial plane to make an emergency landing. REMEMBER –follow airline safety briefing, placard information and cabin/cockpit crew instructions during an in-flight emergency!

While the cabin crew is offering additional safety assurances and briefings, the pilots in the cockpit are talking to air traffic control about the issue, the flight plan, etc. The pilots are communicating on 121.5 MHz, which is the emergency frequency.

Squawking is a radio code that is transmitted by the aircraft to air traffic control. Different squawk codes indicate different identifiers. 7700 is the emergency squawk code.

Post-Emergency Landing Procedures

> ***Stay with the aircraft unless there is an immediate threat to life!***
> Rescue crews will be searching for the aircraft, not you!

In the event of ANY emergency landing of the commercial aircraft, as soon as possible, notify your communications department of the current situation, location and status of yourself, patient and traveling companion. Leave baggage as directed cabin/cockpit crew and provide first aid on an as needed basis

In survival, observe the "Rule Of 3´s". You can survive:
- 3 seconds following a bad decision
- 3 minutes with oxygen
- 3 hours in extreme temperature
- 3 days without water
- 3 weeks without food

Principles of Survival:
- Protection
    - Shelter is priority number 1
- Location
    - Stay close to the aircraft.
- Water
    - If you locate what appears to be clean water, drink it. The risk of dehydration is far worse than the possibility of parasitic infection
- Food
    - Utilize the meal service trays and snack items on the aircraft

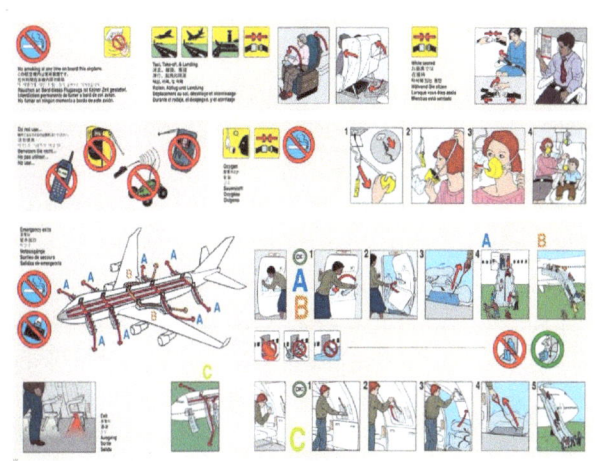

United Airlines

Fire Extinguisher Use

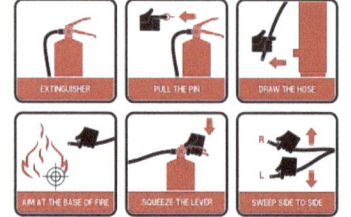

Aircraft with a capacity of greater than 61 must have Halon extinguishers on board.

Per FAA 14 CFR 25.851, there are minimum regulations for the number of extinguishers based on passenger capacity.

Crew Resource Management (CRM)

A non-technical management system that makes optimum use of all available resources (equipment, people, etc.) to promote safety and enhance the efficiency of flight operations.

Human factors control how we do our job. What do we have control over? Interpersonal skills deal with how you interact with other people. Cognitive skills are the mental process like situation awareness, problem solving and decision making. It's primary intention is to enhance communication to avoid errors. In this application, the intention is maximizing all available resources to ensure safety. [3]

HOW DOES THIS APPLY TO WHAT I DO?

Human Factors - Interpersonal & Cognitive Skills
- Communication
    - CRM is more about interpersonal and cognitive skills rather than technical skills.
- Decision making
    - If you aren't making clear, level-headed decisions without first thinking of the outcome, this human factor can lead to severe consequences.
- Situational awareness
    - Referring to you being *AWARE* of what is going on around you. If you don't notice that your patient's foot is in the aisle of the plane. This may result in injury, because you weren't *aware* of what was going on.
- Forward thinking
    - Being able to anticipate future needs– of your patient and how you set up your surroundings for patient care
- Problem solving
    - Unique to the aeromedical transport industry, and medical escorts specifically, is the use of forward thinking to anticipate problems and solutions to those problems.

- Stress management
    - It is important to recognize when you become stressed so you can address it in order to continue to communicate effectively

Human Factors – A Real World Application

You are 8 hours in to a 16 hour transatlantic flight with an uncomplicated post-MI patient. Up until this point, your patient has been without complaints and stable on 2 liters of oxygen via portable oxygen concentrator.

Your patient begins to complain of sudden, crushing chest pain. You manage your patient per your protocols but your patient condition is unchanged. Vitals are HR 130, BP 90/50, RR 28, SpO2 on 4 LPM is 92%. Your patient's skin is cool, clammy and their coloring is gray.

What do you do? How do you manage the situation?

How you approach the cabin crew will demonstrate your ability to manage the situation.

If you are frantic and DEMANDING that the plane makes an emergency landing, you may not be well received. If you are calm, cool and collected - and explain to the cabin crew your concerns, they are more likely to respect your decision making skills.

Another important factor to include in your ability to manage the situation has to do with the contents of the on-board emergency kit that you can utilize to supplement your medical kit. Depending on the airline/routing, the contents of the emergency kit can vary.

Forward Thinking – A Real World Application

You are traveling with your patient from Mauritius Island (MRU) to Frankfurt, Germany (FRA) [MRU-NBO-DOH-FRA] to be evaluated in the cardiac catheterization lab. Your flight from MRU to NBO was delayed 2 hours, meaning you will have missed your connection to NBO. In discussing the situation with airline representatives in MRU, you learn that the next flight from MRU will not depart until the next day.

You find yourself in the patient's pick-up location with no viable way to continue the mission.

How do you manage the situation? In discussing with your program's flight coordinator and client, the decision is made to return the patient to the discharging hospital to await the next practical flights from MRU to FRA.

Not continuing the repatriation, considering the possibility of an extended layover (either in a hotel or new facility), was in the patient's best interest—knowing that the discharge facility and physicians are familiar with the patient and were providing adequate care.

> **While no situation is always black and white, the use of forward thinking to consider possible outcomes is vital in your decision-making process.**

Personal Health & Wellbeing

Your Fitness to Fly

There are many factors that affect your ability to provide safe, competent patient care.
- Acute illness
- Medications
- Alcohol intoxication
- Fatigue or inadequate rest

Circadian Rhythm

Disruption to your circadian rhythm can have internal or external causes.

Internal Causes	External Causes
Medical disorders	Jet lag
Delayed or advanced sleep phase disorder	Shift work

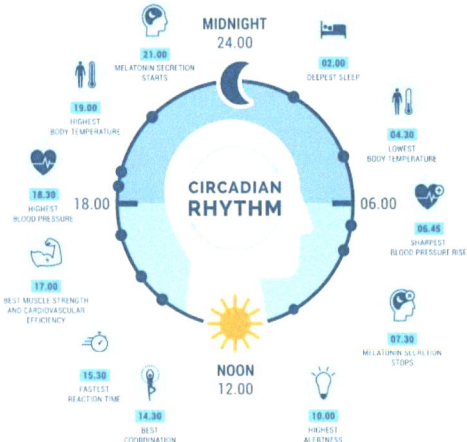

Jet lag is "a temporary disruption of the body's normal biological rhythms after high-speed air travel through several time zones." [4]

Unfortunately, due to the nature of this industry, traveling across multiple time zones is an inevitability. While others may be sleeping on the flight, you are required to remain awake to care for your patient. This compounds, with the potential to cause increased disturbances in your circadian rhythm and sleep-res cycle.

This can and will lead to sleep deprivation, which will impair your decision making skills.

Sleep Inertia

Sleep inertia is defined as a:

"transitional state between sleep and wake, marked by impaired performance, reduced vigilance, and a desire to return to sleep."

 This is an important concept to understand because sleep inertia compounded with jet lag and fatigue can seriously impair your decision making skills, especially after a "cat" nap.

Sleep inertia can last anywhere from 20 to 30 minutes.

Stress Recognition & Management

Stress is the adverse reaction to excessive internal and external pressure and demands placed on a person.

There are two types of stress:
- Eustress is a moderate or normal psychological stress interpreted as being beneficial for the experiencer.
- Distress causes extreme anxiety, sorrow or pain

There are many **causes** of stress, both professional and personal.

Personal/Life
Death of a loved one
End of a relationship
Chronic illness/injury
Emotional problems
Traumatic life events
Caring for family members
Financial
Bullying

Professional
Work overload/too much responsibility
Physical/psychological environment
Poor communication
Lack of career advancement
Loss of a job

There are also many different *manifestations* of stress, both physical and emotional.

Physical Manifestations
Headache
Trouble sleeping or sleeping too much
Muscle pain or tension
Digestive issues
Elevated blood pressure
Change in sex drive

Emotional Manifestations
Feelings of inadequacy
Moodiness
Anxiety
Restlessness
Lack of motivation
Irritability
Depression

Stress Overload

Stress overload can manifest when you pass the 'fatigue' marker on the graphic to the right. The further past optimum stress you are, the more likely are to experience:

- Panic attacks
- Worrying all of the time
- Feeling you're under pressure
- Drinking or using drugs to cope
- Overeating
- Smoking
- Withdrawal from loved ones

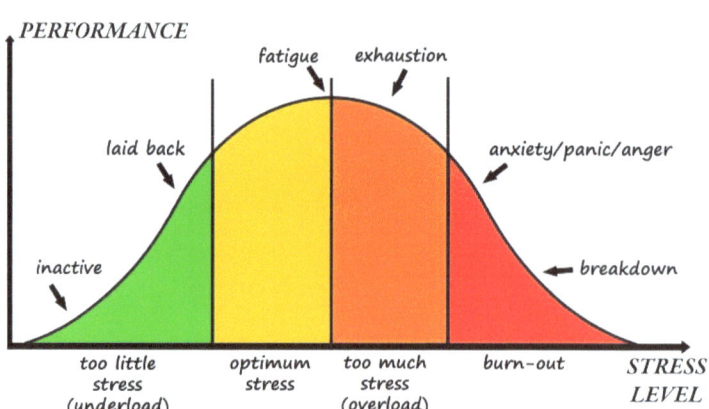

Stress Management

- Accept that some events are out of your control
- Meditation, yoga, tai-chi
- Exercise regularly
- Eat healthy meals
- Work on time management
- Set limits and learn how to say "no" to people
- Make time for hobbies, interests and relaxation
- GET ENOUGH GOOD REST!
- Seek social support and avoid alcohol and drugs
- Seek assistance with a mental health professional if needed
- TAKE A DAY OFF FROM WORK!

Critical Incident Stress Management

CISM is an interventional protocol designed to help deal with major traumatic events. These debriefs are coordinated by your program as needed.

CISM is composed of several portions:
1. Pre-incident education
2. Individual crisis or peer support
3. Demobilization
4. Defusing
5. Debriefing
6. Family support
7. Referral

Fatigue Recognition and Management

Stress, in combination with disruption to your circadian rhythm can and will lead to fatigue.

Fatigue is common in aeromedical transport due to varying work shifts. This is especially true for commercial repatriations that cause jet lag.

Other causes of fatigue include:
- Shift work, especially rotating shifts
- Working long hours
- Prolonged physical or mental activity
- Desynchronized circadian rhythms
- Illness
- Depression/anxiety/stress

Mental Symptoms of Fatigue
Reduced attention span
Forgetfulness
Reduced performance
Impaired judgment and decision making
Irritability/intolerance
Reduced short-term memory
Confusion
Anxiety and social withdrawal
Diminished startle response

Physical Symptoms of Fatigue
Headaches
Muscle aches and pains
Blurred/double vision
Loss of appetite
Decreased motor skills
Tenseness and tremors
Slower reaction times
Falling asleep inappropriately

Fatigue Mitigation
- The first step is recognizing that you are fatigued so you can:
    - Know your alertness pattern
    - Eat nutritionally
    - Get regular exercise
    - Ensure a healthy sleep environment
    - Try to keep a regular schedule
- Respite
    - Can be difficult to manage if you are the sole provider
- Fatigue risk & mitigation self-assessment
- Crew "time out"
    - If the threshold for being able to provide safe and competent care has been exceeded, a time out can be called for safety.
    - This is largely a requirement of accreditation and time outs are reviewed, tracked and trended

Body Mechanics/Safe Lifting

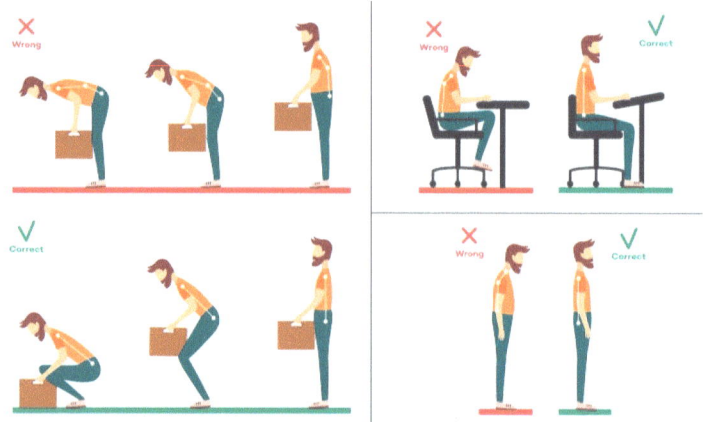

Proper biodynamics of movement helps you avoid muscle fatigue as you walk, bend over, lift objects, or perform other activities of daily living.

This is VITAL when caring for patients so you do not injure yourself!

Patient Transfers

While it is near impossible to review all patient transfer situations, the below video links demonstrate common movements.

Bed to Wheelchair Transfer
(https://www.youtube.com/watch?feature=oembed&v=4BUIu0TNs_8)

Wheelchair to Car Transfer
(https://www.youtube.com/watch?feature=oembed&v=MAoEmnBHPdo)

Infection Control

Bloodborne pathogens are microorganisms such as viruses and bacteria carried in the blood that can cause disease in people who are exposed to those blood containing pathogens.

In the United States, OSHA specifically addresses: Hepatitis B (HBV), Hepatitis C (HCV) and Human Immunodeficiency Virus (HIV). Please refer to your program's infection control policies and procedures for specific details.

Vaccinations

Some vaccines may be required by your program's policies & procedures or to maintain accreditation. They may include:
- Influenza
- Hepatitis A
- Hepatitis B
- Tetanus
- BCG
- Yellow Fever

Always check the WHO recommendations for vaccines prior to accepting an assignment.

Transmission of Bloodborne Diseases

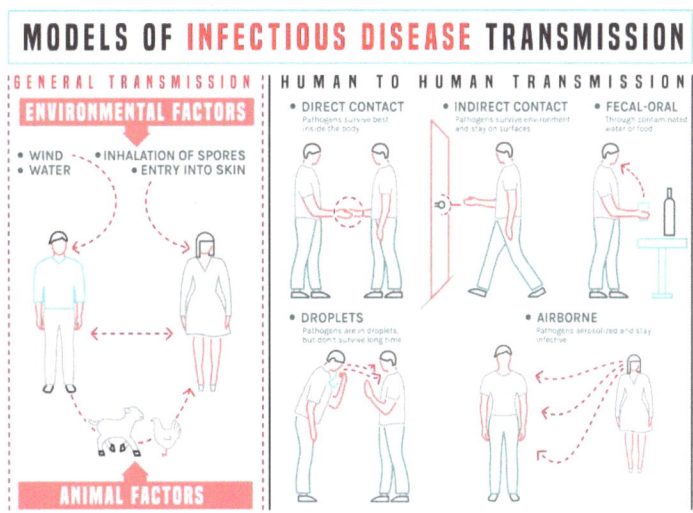

Hepatitis B and Hepatitis C
- Both can be transmitted through blood and bodily fluid.
- HBV can survive in dried blood for 7 days while HCV can survive in dried blood for 4 days.
- There is a vaccine for HBV; no vaccine for HCV.
- In the U.S., HBV vaccine is required to be offered for healthcare workers, they may decline.
- Both can result in long-term liver damage

Human Immunodeficiency Virus
- The virus that causes AIDS
- HIV is spread through blood and bodily fluids
- The virus can be carried for years without detection
- HIV does not live outside of the body for long
- There is no known cure

Infectious Diseases

Include, but are not limited to:
- Tuberculosis
- Viral & Bacterial Meningitis
- Influenza
- SARS
- MERS-CoV
- COVID-19
- Chicken Pox (Varicella)
- Cholera
- Mosquito-borne diseases

Tuberculosis
- Airborne transmission
  - Many countries vaccinate, the U.S. does not
- The TB spore floats in the air until it is inhaled into the lungs
- Active TB can be spread
  - These patients will not be travelling commercially
- Latent TB cannot be spread

Meningitis

Characteristics	Bacterial Meningitis	Viral Meningitis
Treatment	Antibiotics, anti-inflammatories	No specific treatment, treat symptomatically.
Signs/Symptoms	High fever, severe headaches, nausea, vomiting, stiff neck, lethargy, fatigue, photophobia, seizures, purple skin rash	High fever, severe headaches, nausea, vomiting, stiff neck, lethargy, fatigue, photophobia
Complications	Hearing loss, brain damage, learning disability, coma, death	Occur Rarely

Influenza
- Many strains, annual vaccines
    - Flu A (H1N1, H3N2)
    - Flu B (Victoria, Yamagata)
    - Vaccines are updated annually to include the *predicted* strain.
- Droplet precautions
    - Flu infection can evolve to pneumonia, sepsis and death
- While someone may travel with the flu, it is not recommended due to the highly infectious nature of the virus.

SARS & MERS
- Severe Acute Respiratory Syndrome Coronavirus
    - No known cases
- Middle East Respiratory Syndrome Coronavirus
- Cases are rare with a high death rate
- Respiratory illness caused by a strain of the coronavirus

COVID-19
- New strain of coronavirus, easily spread
- Carriers may be asymptomatic and still able to transmit
- Antibodies are short lived (no lifetime immunity)
- At the time of publication, vaccine trials are underway
- Masks that cover the face and nose are utilized worldwide
    - Readily available N95 masks offer a high level of protection from respiratory droplets, while N100 provide the greatest
- PCR testing with lab verified results **_may_** be required prior to travel- depending on the country or countries you will be visiting.

Chicken Pox (Varicella)
- This highly contagious disease spreads through touching or breathing the virus particles that come from blisters or through droplets when an infected person coughs, sneezes, etc.
- Droplet precautions are utilized

Cholera
- "Acute diarrheal infection caused by the ingestion of food or water containing the bacterium Vibrio cholerae" [6]
- Worldwide, there are between 1.3 million to 4.0 million cases every year, with between 21,000 and 143,000 cases.

Mosquito-Borne Diseases
- Transmitted through the bite of a mosquito that is carrying the virus from an infected person.
- Not transmitted through coughing, sneezing, etc.
- Spreads quickly in areas without mosquito control and when bug repellent is not used.
- When travelling to tropical locations, bring bug spray for your protection
- There are many different mosquito-borne diseases, some lead to hemorrhage and shock (Dengue Fever, West Nile Virus).
- Malaria and Zika are also prevalent

Antibiotic Resistant Bacteria

If transporting a patient with an antibiotic resistant infection, it is important to understand there are more and more frequent infections caused by resistant bacteria. Ensure you utilize appropriate personal protective equipment for the task, like dressing changes and containing bodily fluids.

Personal Protective Equipment

Remember: for commercial repatriations with the general population, your patient will most likely NOT be transported if they are infectious/contagious.

- Universal precautions
    - Assume that all blood and bodily fluids contains pathogens
- Gloves
    - Used for all patient contacts
- Goggles
    - Used when there is a possibility of bodily fluid splash
- Masks
    - Chance of droplet or body fluid splash
- Gowns
    - To be worn when there is a possibility of bodily fluid splash on your clothing

 CDC Guidelines on Personal Protective Equipment
https://www.cdc.gov/infectioncontrol/guidelines/isolation/appendix/type-duration-precautions.html

Infection Control

- Aircraft air circulation [10]
    - Aircraft air is circulated from bottom to top, through HEPA filters roughly two dozen times per hour. Air is EXCHANGED from the inside to the outside approximately 12 times per hour
- Handwashing
    - Most vital aspect of infection control. Use of alcohol based hand sanitizer is acceptable when soap and water are not available
- Frequent disinfection of work areas and patient contact surfaces
- Sharps disposal in appropriate container
- Soiled materials disposal in appropriately marked bags

If you are exposed to an infectious disease, the most important thing you can do is STAY CALM and assess the situation. Notify your manager as soon as reasonably possible.

Conclusion

You are the only person responsible for your personal health and wellbeing, especially when conducting air medical transport. Do not fly while acutely ill to prevent fatigue and potential spread to other individuals.

Circadian rhythm disturbances can lead to stress and fatigue. Recognition is vital and proper methods to mitigate stress and fatigue will help you in the future.

Proper body mechanics will help you avoid painful injuries. Appropriate PPE should be used and excellent hand hygiene is imperative! Airlines will provide the medical clearance to fly; an infectious patient will most likely NOT be travelling commercially.

COMMERCIAL TRANSPORT ENVIRONMENT

Mission Planning & Following

Logistics & Communication Department

- Quote acceptance and confirmation of the medical escort staff
    - Confirmation of medical report/condition
    - Medical clearance, including oxygen (if needed)
- Confirm patient pick-up and drop-off locations
- Review patient and passenger luggage
- Airline ticketing
- Booking of hotels
- Confirmation of ground transport
- Risk assessment

<u>The communications department is your main point of contact with your program and the client.</u>

Mission Tracking & PAIP

- Flight following takes place 24/7/365 via commercially available programs, allowing the communications department to provide updates to the client, ground transport etc.
    - Especially useful in the event of delays
- Post-Accident/Incident Plan (PAIP)
    - In the event of an overdue or missing aircraft, no communication from the clinician, your program may have a PAIP in place
    - Provides guidance to management on alternate attempts to locate the clinician and notifications.

Ground Transport Operations

Ground Transport without a patient could be:
- Pre-arranged car
- Rideshare
- Taxi

Refer to your program's safety policies regarding the use of certain modes of transport without the patient.

Ground Ambulance
- Need due to mobility, clinical status, amount of luggage or vehicle availability
- Safety
    - Remain seated and seat belted at all times. All equipment and luggage is to be secured
- Stretcher and vehicle operation
    - Responsibility of ambulance crew ONLY
- Lights and sirens
    - Strongly discouraged due to inherent danger

Town Car/Limo/SUV

Not every patient you transfer will require a ground ambulance. It is common to utilize a town car or SUV for transport. These patients are able to sit upright and should only require minimal assistance in and out of the vehicle.

Careful consideration for the type of patient. *Example*: a patient with a repaired hip may do better with a car instead of an SUV because it requires less weight bearing to step up and in. When you are at the bedside for your pre-flight, confirm the mode of transport that has been booked. This ties into the forward thinking as part of CRM

Considerations:

- Is the vehicle low to the ground? Will they be able to get in and out?
- Is the vehicle too high up? Are they able to lift their leg up and in?

Wheelchair Assistance

Frequently, a *porter* will assist you and your patient through the airport to the lounge or departure gate. Keep in mind that depending on the airport, they may have different loading procedures like carry on board or Ambu-lift.

Wheelchair assistance is divided into 3 categories:
- WCHR (R=Ramp)
    - Wheelchair to the aircraft ramp. Passenger is able to use stairs and ambulate in the cabin.
- WCHS (S=Stairs)
    - Passenger cannot climb stairs, a high-lift may be utilized to lift the patient on to the plane or they may be carried by ground personnel
- WCHC (C=Cabin)
    - Passenger is unable to ambulate to their seat. Aisle chair will be required.

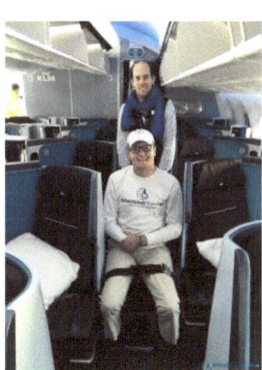

You will find if your patient requires more or less assistance than is booked on their reservation, you will be able to work with the airline and ground crews to ensure they receive the appropriate level of assistance.

While at the Airport
- Security
    - Assist your patient with luggage and personal items
    - Be aware that certain medications or medical supplies are forbidden in certain countries or regions. Your supervisor or flight coordinator should inform you. However, it is best to conduct your own due diligence to ensure that you are not in possession of anything that could land you in police custody.
- Lounge
    - If available and time permitting, a nice place to relax and have a snack prior to your flight
- Departure Gate
    - Confirm with the airline representative that seats are together
- Restroom
    - Much easier to utilize the restroom in the terminal than on the aircraft
- Meals
    - Offer your patient and/or travel companion a meal or drink, time permitting.

Flight Physiology & Stressors of Transport

Contraindications/Considerations to commercial transport:
- Hgb <8.0
    - Oxygen binding ability
- Trapped air inside of the body
    - Gaseous expansion
- Use of oxygen (at sea level) >4 LPM
    - Most oxygen delivery devices do not offer delivery greater than 4 LPM

Basic Flight Terminology
- Above Ground Level (AGL)
- Above Sea Level (ASL)
- Mean Sea Level (MSL)

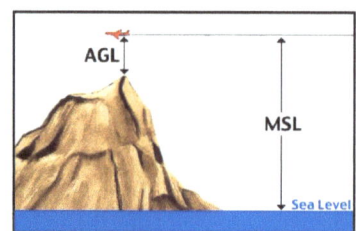

Atmospheric Composition
- Three gases constitute 99% of the atmosphere
- Nitrogen: 78%
- Oxygen: 21%
- Argon: 0.93%
- Same composition at 1000', 5000', 25,000'

Barometric Pressure Values
Weight of air, may be expressed in torr or mmHg

Sea Level	760 torr	(1 ATM)
10k ft. MSL	523 torr	
18k ft. MSL	380 torr	(1/2 ATM)
63k ft. MSL	0 torr	(0 ATM)

Altitude Zones
- Physiologic Zone- Sea Level to 10k MSL
    - Reduction in night vision at 5,000 MSL
- Physiologically Deficient Zone- 10k to 50k MSL
    - 10,000ft MSL = PaO2 61mmHg (85-90% SpO2)
- Space Equivalent Zone- > 50K MSL

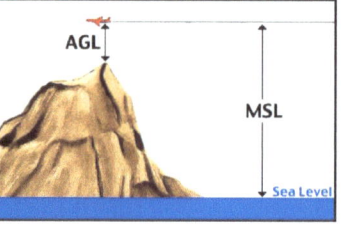

Physiologically Deficient Zone
- This is where commercial travel takes place
- In the commercial cabin when a sudden decompression occurs, Time of Useful Consciousness (TUC) is cut in half

- A sign of depressurization is cooler temperatures in the cabin and fogging windows
- Normally 90 seconds of useful consciousness at 30,000 ft.
    - If a rapid decompression occurs, TUC is now around 45 sec

Simulated altitude of 45,000' with rapid depressurization
https://www.youtube.com/watch?v=6EfvI6AwILo

Gas Laws

Boyle's Law: The pressure of a gas is inversely proportional to the volume of a gas at a constant temperature. Think "Boyle's Balloon" – a balloon gets bigger the higher it goes due to the outside pressure decreasing and inside pressure increasing.

As altitude increases, atmospheric pressure decreases
$$P_1V_1 = P_2V_2$$

Dalton's Law: "Law of partial pressures." The total pressure of a gas mixture is the sum of the partial pressures of all the gases in the mixture.

Same amount of gas molecules, just further apart

As altitude increases, there is less partial pressure but the same concentration of gasses. This allows for hypoxia and soft tissue swelling.

Other Gas Laws

Charles' Law: The volume of gas is directly proportional to the temperature
As air heats up, molecules spread and make air less dense

Fick's Law: Diffusion of gas is:
- Proportional to the difference in partial pressure
- Proportional to the area of the membrane
- Inversely proportional to the thickness of the membrane

Henry's Law: The quantity of gas dissolved in 1 cm^3 (1 mL) of a liquid is proportional to the partial pressure of the gas in contact with the liquid.

Example: Henry's Heineken (when you open a bottle or can of a carbonated drink, there is gas released.

Altitude Effects

The commercial aircraft cabin is pressurized between 5,000' and 8,000' (Aerospace Medical Association).

- A cold, dry, high altitude environment has the greatest negative effect on your patient!
- Every 1,000 foot increase in elevation causes temperatures to drop 2° C

Barodontalgia
- Occurs on Ascent
- Air trapped in fillings expands due to Boyle's law
- Also referred to as "Aerodontalgia"

Barotitis Media
- Occurs on Descent
- Most common trapped-gas problem
- Eustachian Tube Dysfunction, also known as "ear block"

Barosinusitis
- Can occur on BOTH Ascent (32%) and Descent (68%)
- Can also cause pain in the maxillary teeth
- "Sinus Block"

Decompression Sickness
- Henry's law
- Nitrogen bubbles form at one or more locations within the body
- Normally excess nitrogen diffuses into the capillaries in a solution
- Rapid decrease in pressure causes nitrogen to leave as a gas
- Type I: seen and felt in the skin
- Type II: neurologic symptoms, hypovolemic shock

Primary Stressors of Flight

All of the following issues, in combination with circadian rhythm disruption, stress, etc. can lead to increased fatigue.
- Decreased levels of PO2
- Barometric Pressure Changes
    - Greatest pressure changes occur from sea level to 5,000 feet
- Thermal Changes
    - Decreased humidity
    - Noise
    - Increased patient anxiety
    - Fatigue
    - Spatial disorientation and illusions of flight – not very often as a commercial passenger!
    - Fuel Vapors, other odors
    - Gravitational Forces
    - Vibration- increased metabolism and oxygen demand
        - Roadway
        - Turbulence
        - Aircraft

Self-imposed stressors are those that we have direct control over. These can affect both you and your patient. These include:
- Dehydration
- Exhaustion
- Alcohol
- Tobacco
- Hypoglycemia

Types Of Hypoxia

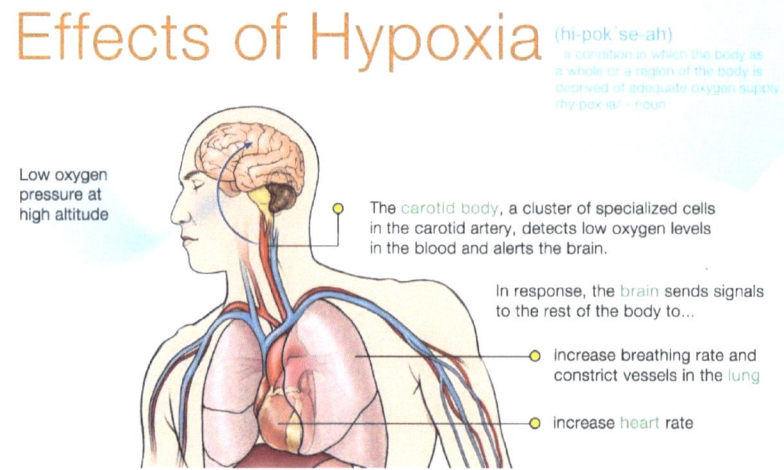

Hypoxic
- "Not enough oxygen in the air"
- Decreased partial pressure of oxygen at altitude
- Deficiency in alveolar O2 exchange
- Cardiovascular/Pneumothorax patients are more susceptible to this type of hypoxia
- Hypoxia at the lung level

Stagnant
- "Blood isn't moving"
- High G-forces
- Blood pooling
- Cardiogenic shock
- Sitting with legs in a dependent position
- Reduced cardiac output
- Hypoxia at the circulatory level

Hypemic
- Also known as Anemic Hypoxia
- Anemia, CO poisoning, Sickle Cell
- Reduction in the O2 carrying capacity of blood
- Hypoxia at the blood level

Histotoxic
- "Poisoning"
- Plenty of O2 available
- Tissues cannot accept
- Cyanide, Alcohol, Sodium Nitroprusside (Nipride)
- Hypoxia at the cellular level

Stages of Hypoxia "ICDC"
- **I**ndifferent (most important)
    - Full reasoning abilities
    - Some loss of night vision
- **C**ompensated
    - Increased HR and ventilations
    - Slowed judgement
- **D**isturbance
    - Appears drunk
    - Loss of cognitive abilities and fine motor skills
- **C**ritical
    - Unconsciousness
    - Brain damage
    - Death

Gravitational Pulls - Effects on Crew & Patients
- G-forces cause blood pressure to drop
- People most affected by high G-forces
    - On BP meds (especially Beta Blockers)
    - Dehydrated
- Gx = Anterior/Posterior
    - Best tolerated
- Accelerating for take-off and initial climb cause positive G-forces, and they are in the "Gx" axis

Medical Equipment, Oxygen, Classes Of Travel & Stretchers

Medical Equipment
- Pulse Oximeter
- Blood Pressure Cuff
- Glucometer
- Portable Oxygen Concentrator (POC)

Pulse dose vs. continuous flow
(https://www.youtube.com/watch?feature=oembed&v=PNDEYQdRH8o)

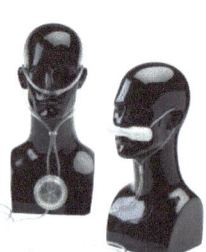

- o Pulse dose oxygen could require you to coach your patient on synchronizing their breath with the POC
- o How much oxygen is your patient currently receiving?
  - Refer to your program's protocols on the use of an Oxymizer to create a reservoir and increase oxygen saturations on low flow
  - Some experienced medical escorts will "double up" on oxygen—POC and airline tanks.
- o Examples of POCs:
  - Inogen
  - Airsep
  - Respironics
- Airline Provided Oxygen
  - o Airline oxygen may be arranged ahead of time. You attach a nasal cannula to the airline oxygen tank and swap tanks when empty. The cabin crew will assist you with this. This oxygen is typically delivered by pulse dose with varying liter flows (0-15 LPM vs. 2 or 4 LPM only).
  - o Please note that some airline oxygen bottles come with a mask or cannula attached. If you there is no delivery device attached, you *may* require an attachment for your standard device to work with the bottle.

Liron Beltzer, M.D.

Classes of Service

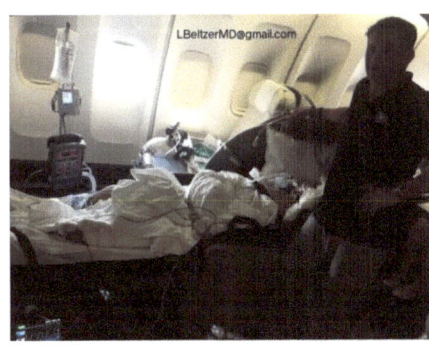

Business or First Class
- Patients that are able to sit up for taxi, take-off and landing
- Depending on airline, seats may recline to near flat or may convert to a fully flat bed.
- Please note that complex patients *may* be transferred in the business or first-class cabin with airline approval.

Economy
- Typically utilized for non-medical patients or those with a behavioral/psychiatric diagnosis
- Stretchers
  - Stretcher transfers have their own challenges. It can be difficult to access your patient in the event of resuscitation. They also offer limited privacy for the patient and no amenities such as entertainment, food options, etc.

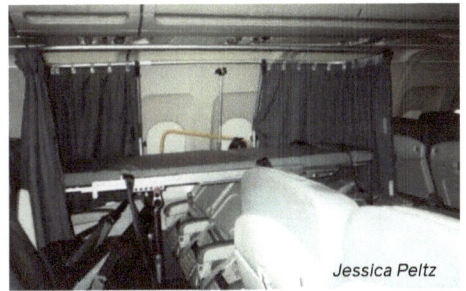

- Stretcher Patients
  - Basic
    - Orthopedic injury/surgery
    - Non-ambulatory
  - Advanced/Critical
    - Cardiac monitoring, vasoactive drips, sedation, ventilators

Loading of Stretcher Patients
- Commercial stretcher patients will not be ambulating on or off the aircraft.
- Ambu-Lift
- Carry on board

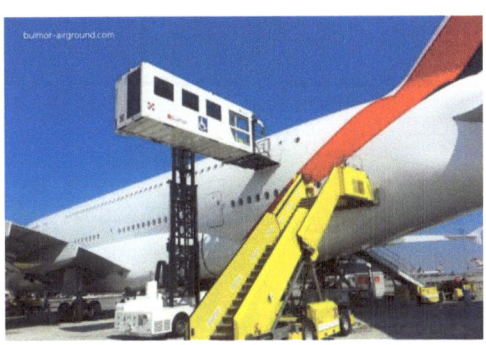
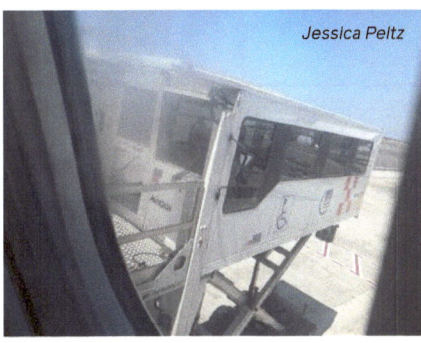
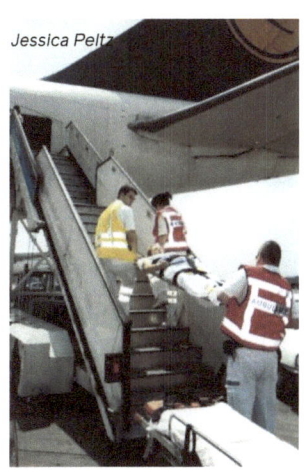

In-Flight Management

Use of Forward Thinking

- Assessment
    - Confirm the patient's fitness to fly commercially. Your assessment may discover a contraindication to commercial transport!
- Preparation
    - Luggage packed, needed items in carry on, patient dressed appropriately, passports in-hand
    - Ensure that any items the patient may need are in a carry-on. This may include medications, cellular phone, books, glasses, etc.
    - In the event that travel planning was unable to seat you together, speak to the counter or gate agent-- especially for a seat close to the restroom if your patient will require it (continent, no urinary catheter). *This is an effective way to practice your forward thinking skills.*
    - *Of vital importance is seating. Are the seats in closed off suites or open? This ties into your ability to visualize, monitor and treat your patient.*
        - Avoid bulkheads when possible. While they may offer more leg room, you will not be able to administer oxygen via POC until after 10,000' due to no seat in front of you.
        - While your CHF patient may be comfortable laying fully flat, consider the most APPROPRIATE positioning for the flight- your patient could end up with an exacerbation!
        - Consider the G-Forces and clinical picture regarding seat position (forward or rear facing). This may tie into nausea/vomiting with air sickness.

- Treatment
    - Using discretion while providing care to your patient can be difficult. This may include measuring vital signs, changing POC batteries, administering medications, assisting them with transfers and to the restroom, etc.
- Handling
    - Use of assistive devices (wheelchair, walker, you)
    - Moving about the aircraft cabin with a mobility impaired individual can be challenging. Larger aircraft have an on-board wheelchair and a handicap restroom.
- Equipment
    - What do you anticipate needing for your flight? POC batteries? Medications? Vitals sign tools?
    - Where will you place everything you need? Are they easily accessible from your carry on? If you are in business or first, you will have some storage areas. If you are in economy seating or stretcher, you will have to ensure that you can easily access your supplies.

Work Area & Resources

- Patient acuity
    - The higher the acuity, the more difficult it can be to provide care. This is outside of a typical/routine work environment. Being able to function without a dedicated workspace, or to not be able to get up without putting your tray table away can take some acclimation.
    - We learned through crew resource management the importance of forward thinking.
- Work environment
    - In commercial transport, if you do not have it with you on the plane, you're not going to have it. Make sure to bring all anticipated supplies and equipment with you. There are limited resources on-board-- you can't just run to the supply closet or access another medical bag for an item.
    - Use a pressure bag to administer IV fluids when you are unable to hang them.
- Available resources
    - Depending on your program's scope of practice, you may have your patient on continuous cardiac monitoring, oxygen and IV medications while in business or first class. Some may require bolus enteral feeds. Keep in mind, some of these longer transports exceed 12 hours!
    - Electrical outlets are available on the aircraft. Consider an inverter and extension cord to power your POC, with the cooperation of the cabin crew.
- Appropriate medications & batteries for your transport
    - At a minimum, you should have 48 hours' worth of the patient's medications with you in the event of a flight delay or cancellation. This should be requested at the initiation of the mission or upon your arrival at the discharging facility.
    - The airlines require that you have 1.5x the anticipated battery needs for a POC. You should be able to plug the POC in at the airport to charge/maintain batteries, but *do not rely on being able to use the aircraft power!*

Prevention of DVT/VTE

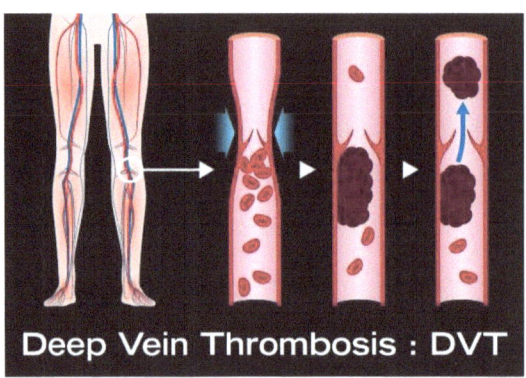

Deep Vein Thrombosis (DVT) and Venous Thromboembolism (VTE) are a real risk of air travel
- A clot in the leg can dislodge and travel to the lungs, causing a pulmonary embolism.
- Risk factors
    - How long is your flight?
    - Age > 40
    - Obesity
    - Surgery or injury withing 3 months
    - Use of estrogen containing contraceptives or hormone replacement therapy
    - Pregnancy/postpartum
    - History of blood clots
    - Active cancer or recent treatment
    - Limited mobility
    - Large vessel vascular access
    - Varicose veins
- What can I do for my patient?
    - Pharmacology (SQ Heparin or LMWH, ASA)
    - Compression stockings
    - Ambulation or in-seat exercises [8]

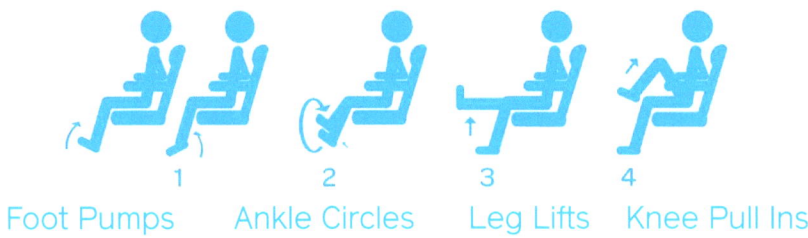

Prevention of Skin Breakdown

If your patient has altered sensorium (due to strokes or diseases like Alzheimer's or Dementia), they may not be able to

1. Reposition themselves to prevent skin breakdown or
2. Feel when their position needs to be changed.

As the medical escort, it is your duty to ensure that your patient is repositioned for comfort and skin integrity no less than every two hours. This applies to all patients in all classes of travel.

 This is especially important if your patient has impaired skin integrity PRIOR to the mission. While it can be difficult to reposition your patient in the limited working environment, utilize extra pillows and blankets to provide additional pressure offloading or to aid in turning.

- Limited mobility
- Skin moisture (sweat, use of diapers)
- Inadequate pressure relief
- Can lead to impaired skin integrity
- Infection
- Prolonged healing

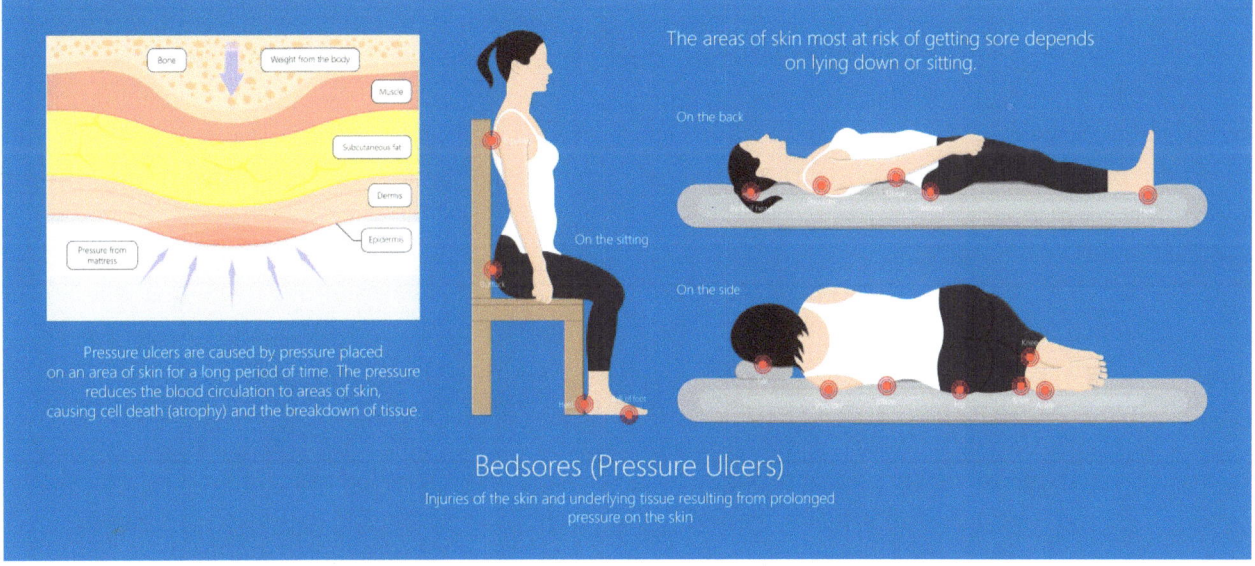

Putting it all Together

- Confirmation
    - You will be confirmed for the mission and provided preliminary medical information, airline and hotel confirmations, as well as any mission specific items.
- Call for medical report
    - Per your programs policies & procedures, an updated medical report should be obtained to confirm the patient's suitability for commercial transfer.
- Communicate!
    - Per your programs policies & procedures
- Arrival in patient location city
    - You may be asked to visit the patient in person (depending on your arrival time) to discuss travel plans and perform a physical assessment.
    - Get some rest at your hotel!
- Transport day

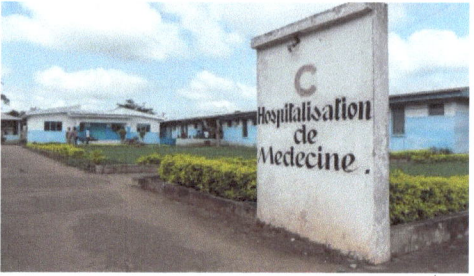

    - Ground transport will have most likely been set up by your program. Be sure to confirm that transport times are appropriate for the distance to the airport, as well as the time needed to arrive..
    - Perform another quick assessment, load all luggage in transport and depart for the airport
- Arrival at the airport
    - Depending on your patient's mobility, proceed to the check-in counter with their passport or ID and retrieve a wheelchair. At this time, confirm seating is together and close to the restroom if needed. If you have oxygen, also confirm that it is on the reservation. A porter will most likely assist you through the airport.
    - If time permits and one is available, proceed to the business/first class lounge for comfort.
- Boarding the plane
    - You will be boarding the plane first. If your patient requires the aisle chair, ground personnel will operate it. Stay with your patient throughout this process.
    - For stretchers, ground ambulance crews and/or airline ground crew will coordinate and direct the loading process for your patient. This begins at the check-in counter. Once they are on board, confirm that they are secured to the stretcher and comfortable.
    - Ensure your patient is secured in the aircraft seat and luggage is stowed.

- Stretcher transfers
    - Stretcher transfers are more logistically complicated. Luggage still needs to be obtained and customs still needs to be cleared. You will rely on the direction of the ground personnel at the arrival airport.

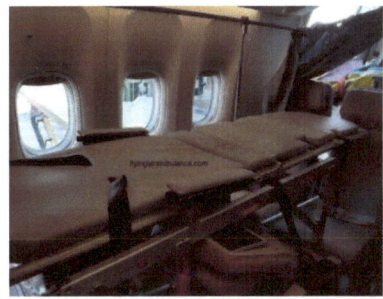

- In-flight
    - While in-flight, you are to attend to your patient's needs and assist them in any way they need it, including dietary restrictions. If they have new complaints, treat per protocol.
- Layovers
    - You will be the last off of the plane. If you have a tight connection, notify the cabin crew so arrangements can be made to assist you to your next gate.

- Missed flights
    - This is a very stressful situation for all involved. After notifying your communications/logistics department, there is a high probability that you will be able to rebook faster and easier than the travel department. Discuss your options with airline representatives.
    - Confer with your point of contact to determine the best way to move forward.
- Arrival destination city
    - Obtain checked bags and rendezvous with pre-arranged ground transportation.
    - More likely than not, you will accompany your patient to their final destination of home or medical facility. Leave a record of transport when turning care over.
- Mission complete
    - At this point, depending on where you live and where you delivered your patient, you will return home, to a hotel or to the airport.

Conclusion

You will be confirmed for the mission, provided preliminary medical information, airline and hotel confirmations, as well as any mission specific items. Per your programs policies & procedures, an updated medical report should be obtained to confirm the patient's suitability for commercial transfer.

Communicate per your program's policies & procedures. You may be asked to visit the patient in person (depending on your arrival time) to discuss travel plans and perform a physical assessment.

Get some rest at your hotel to help mitigate potential fatigue.

Ground transport will have most likely have been set up by your program. Be sure to confirm that times are appropriate for your travel distance to the airport. Perform another quick assessment, prepare all luggage for transport and head to the airport

CLINICAL GUIDELINES AND EMERGENCIES

 A brief note: Regardless of your patient's age, diagnosis, or current clinical status, anticipating their clinical picture (forward thinking) is vital for patient care. For example, if your patient becomes tachycardic during take-off, take a moment to run through some differential diagnoses before administering beta blockers. It is likely that they were a little nervous during take-off and will then have some bradycardia due to the beta blocker.

Disaster & Triage

System of prioritizing patients based on injury severity. In the commercial environment, these principles will generally NOT apply to you. However, if you are involved in an emergency landing, you may need to apply this information immediately upon making contact with the ground.

- START triage
    - Simple Triage and Rapid Treatment
- JumpSTART (Pediatrics, under the age of 8)

The following are applied:
- Immediate (red)
- Delayed (yellow)
- Minimal (green)
- Expectant (black or zebra)

Activating a Medical Emergency Onboard

This is one of the worst things a medical escort professional can think of. Keeping *calm* is vital. This allows you to use your experience to treat your patient.

The decision to make an emergency landing is made by the captain of the aircraft. There are many considerations when making that decision—aircraft location, duration of time remaining on intended flight, medical advice from MedAire/MedLink, Stat-MD, etc.

MedAire/MedLink and STAT-MD are physician consultant programs for the aviation sector. They can be reached with the facilitation of the aircraft captain. Among other services, they provide clinical guidance in the event of a medical emergency on board.

Airlines have their own protocols/procedures for how to move forward in these circumstances– guidance/recommendations from YOU *may* not be considered– but advice from MedAire/MedLink and STAT-MD *most likely will be*.

Regardless-- it is imperative that you provide the best care for your patient that you can with the *resources* you have. Once you notify the cabin crew of the medical emergency, you may find yourself surrounded by willing volunteers to help. Per your programs policies, you may take directives from an on-board physician. If speaking directly to the MedAire/MedLink physician, you may follow those orders.

Patient Medical Emergency
- Recognize the need for intervention
- Treat within your protocols
- Notify cabin crew
- Onboard emergency kit
- Other licensed passengers
- MedAire/MedLink

Please note that some airlines will not permit you to access the onboard medical kit without producing a professional license.

The contents of the emergency kit can vary from airline to airline, and can be determined by flight locations as well (within Africa alone versus departing from the U.S.). This is determined by the governing aviation authority for the country or continent.

You can expect to see: a BVM, epinephrine, BP cuff, stethoscope, naloxone, antacids, aspirin. Refer to "'Is there a doctor on board?': Practical recommendations for managing in-flight medical emergencies".

Anatomy & Physiology – 'Special Populations'

We will briefly review some basic material regarding pregnancy, neonates and the pediatric population.

Physiologic Changes During Pregnancy

Flying during pregnancy is generally accepted as safe. Those after 36 weeks may need their obstetrician to provide documentation stating they are FTF.

Cardiovascular
- Cardiac output increases 20-40%
- Increased plasma and decreased vascular resistance
- Increase in pulse by 10-15 bpm
    - Must be considered when interpreting a tachycardia response to hypovolemia
- Blood pressure decreases 10-15 Systolic
- ECG changes
    - Axis deviation shift
    - Inverted T waves

Blood volume and composition changes
- Increased plasma and erythrocytes
- Hematocrit value decreases
    - Due to increase in total plasma, offering a relative anemia
- Elevated leukocytes
- Increased serum albumin
- Increased clotting factors
    - DVT Risk increased
        - Especially coupled with immobility during flying

Respiratory changes
- Increased rate and minute volume
    - Lower PCO2 ≈ 30mmHg
    - pH ranging from 7.40-7.47
- Increased oxygen demand by fetus means supplemental oxygen should be considered

GI System
- Delayed GI emptying increases risk for aspiration
- Endocrine
    - Increased risk of insulin resistance

Pregnancy Terms
- Preterm- before 38 weeks
- Full term 38-42 weeks
- Post term- after 42 weeks
- Consider GTPAL assessment
    - Gravida
    - Term births
    - Preterm births
    - Abortions
    - Living children

General Assessments
- Place patient in the left lateral recumbent position
    - Check temperature
    - Potential for sepsis
        - Early treatment with Ampicillin and Gentamicin
- Blood pressure
    - Pregnancy Induced Hypertension, pre-eclampsia, eclampsia
- Oxygen saturations

Anatomy and Physiology of the Neonate

Neonates are obligate nasal breathers and their large occiput can cause the tongue to obstruct the airway.

- Thermoregulatory issues
    - High body surface area to body weight ratio
    - Limited subcutaneous fat stores
- Respiratory function and structure
    - Anatomical features
        - Cricoid ring is the narrowest part
    - Surfactant deficiency
    - High oxygen demand
- Cardiovascular
- Heart rate between 120-160
- Newborns go through significant changes after their first breath
- Decrease in pulmonary vascular resistance
- Closure of foramen ovale
- Decrease of flow through ductus arteriosus

Anatomy and Physiology of the Pediatric Patient

- Limited duration of compensatory mechanisms
- Lower airways are smaller, therefore more prone to obstruction and collapse
- Tend to have highly reactive airways
- Higher risk of aspiration
- Differences in skull anatomy and brain development
    - Higher chance of TBI due to lack of compartmentalization and more room in the skull
- Bones are not fully calcified
- Abdominal muscles are not fully developed
    - Increased risk of splenic fracture or lacerated liver
    - Liver function is immature, with few glucose stores and prolonged clotting time
- Increased renal function
    - Infant: 2mL/kg/hr, pediatric: 1mL/kg/hr UOP
- Pediatric metabolism operates at a higher rate than adults

Pediatric Assessment Triangle
- Appearance: "TICLS" (tickles)
    - Tone
    - Interactiveness
    - Consolability
    - Look or gaze
    - Speech or cry
- Work of Breathing
- Circulation

Pediatric Vitals
- Heart rate will be dependent on age
- Blood pressure can be estimated with the following formulas:
    - Normotensive Systolic BP: 90 + 2 (age in years)
    - Hypotensive Systolic BP: 70 + 2 (age in years)

It is important to note, a child may lose up to 25-30% of their total volume before hypotension is noted. Estimated circulating blood volume is 80mL/kg of body weight.

Blood replacement is estimated at 10mL/kg of body weight, while fluid resuscitation is below:
- Emergent fluid resuscitation
    - 20mL/kg
    - Limit to 2 boluses before considering blood products

Maintenance fluids:

    First 1-10 kg   4 mL/kg/hr
    (10kg x 4 mL = 40 mL)

    second 10-20 kg   2 mL/kg/hr
    (10kg x 2 mL = 20 mL)

    Weight >20 kg   1 mL/kg/hr

Shortcut method:

    If patient is over 20kg, 40 + weight in kg will give you the same result

    Example for a 25 kg child:.

(10 kg x 4 mL = 40 mL) + (10 kg x 2 mL = 20 mL) + (5 kg x 1 mL = 5 mL) = **65 mL/hr**

Pediatric Emergencies

Croup
- Viral infection that most often affects the larynx
- Usually not life threatening
- Gradual onset with URI, low grade fever
- "Barking seal" cough that becomes worse at night
- Most common under the age of 3
- Treat with humidified O2, racemic epinephrine and steroids

Epiglottitis
- Bacterial infection
- Life threatening
    - Drooling, dysphagia, dysphonia, distress
- Rapid onset fever, stridor
- Keep the child calm due to possible rapid airway loss

Bronchiolitis
- Swelling of the bronchiole walls
- Usually not life threatening
- >90% viral - Respiratory Syncytial Virus
    - Highly contagious and isolation is required
- Cough, shortness of breath, nasal flaring, wheezing/crackling on exam

Pediatric Trauma
- TBI is the leading cause of morbidity and mortality in children
    - Higher risk of subdural hematoma
- 70-80% of all pediatric deaths from trauma
- Most common source is motor vehicle crashes
- Less common: sports, falls, abuse
- Concussions
- Peds at high risk for SCIWORA (spinal cord injury without radiographic abnormalities)

Adult Emergencies

Neurological & Neurosurgical Emergencies

Anatomy of the skull
- Superior surfaces form a smooth inner wall
- Basilar skull contains many ridges and folds with sharp edges

Neurological Exam
- Mental and emotional status
- Glasgow Coma Scale
- Cranial nerve assessments

Glasgow Coma Scale
- Minor Injury: 13-15
- Moderate Injury: 9-12
- Severe Injury: <8

Cranial Nerve Assessments
- Follow the pen
- Pupillary response
- Observing the patient swallow
- Shrug shoulders
- Etc.

GLASGOW COMA SCALE	
EYE OPENING RESPONSE	Spontaneous — 4
	To sound — 3
	To pressure — 2
	None — 1
VERBAL RESPONSE	Orientated — 5
	Confused — 4
	Words — 3
	Sounds — 2
	None — 1
MOTOR RESPONSE	Obey commands — 6
	Localising — 5
	Normal flexion — 4
	Abnormal flexion — 3
	Extension — 2
	None — 1

Meningeal Irritation
- Most commonly associated with Meningitis
    - Caused by infection, treated based on cause
        - Bacterial, viral, fungal, parasitic, or other toxins
- Disease is carried in the cerebral spinal fluid (CSF)
- Use standard PPE (gloves, mask, gown)
- Signs include:
    - Generalized throbbing, progressing headache
    - Photophobia
    - Nuchal rigidity

Kernig's Sign: Severe stiffness of the hamstrings causes an inability to straighten the leg when the hip is flexed to 90 degrees ("Kicking Kernig's")

Brudzinski's Sign: the appearance of involuntary lifting of the legs when lifting a patient's head with the patient

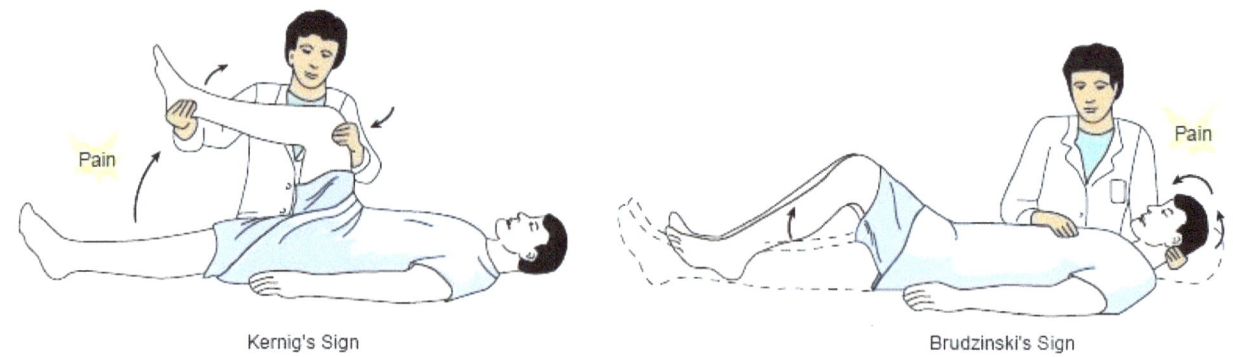

Testing for meningeal irritation. (A) Kernig's sign. (B) Brudzinski's sign.

Brain Injuries

Caused by trauma to the head, your patient will be stabilized before commercial transport. It is important to understand the mechanisms behind the insult to the brain and what to look for in your patient. We are going to briefly go over some medications that are often used in the treatment of head injuries.

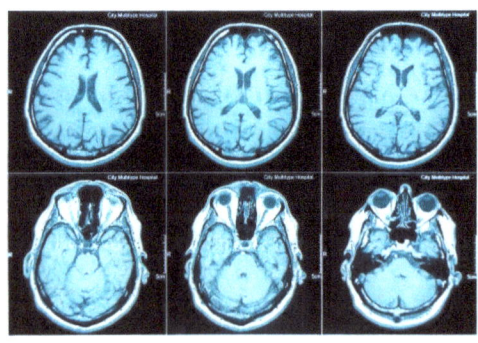

Normal Brain Imaging

Head Trauma can lead to:
- Bleeding within the brain
- Bleeding within the protective layers of the skull
    - Transport considerations: patient may have a drain in place
- Injuries not visible on imaging

Subdural & Epidural Hematomas

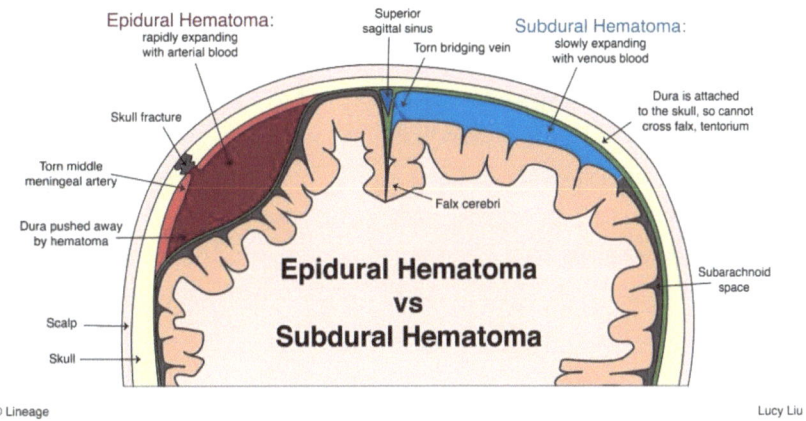

Epidural Hematoma
- Described as lenticular in shape
- Most are arterial in nature, as a result of a blow to the temporal region and concomitant disruption of the middle meningeal artery
- Loss of consciousness followed by a lucid interval
- May last minutes to hours
- Secondary rapid deterioration of consciousness

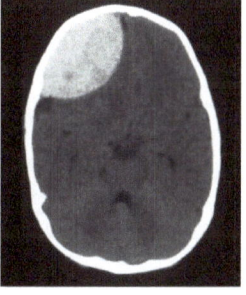

Subdural Hematoma
- "Venous Lakes"
- Tearing of the bridging veins to the subdural space
- Six times more common than epidural with a higher mortality
- Elderly and children highly susceptible
- Intraventricular hemorrhage has increased mortality
- Types:
  - Acute
    - Signs/symptoms appear within 24 hours of injury
    - Often seen with acceleration-deceleration injuries
  - Subacute
    - Signs/symptoms appear between 2 days and 2 weeks
  - Chronic
    - Signs/symptoms appear after 2 weeks

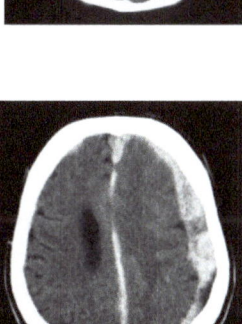

Sub Arachnoid Hemorrhage
- "Worst headache of my life"
- Starfish Pattern on CT
- Avoid lumbar punctures until CT scan complete
- Keep systolic BP below 140mmHg
- Treatment:
    - Treat with Nimodipine (Nimotop)
        - Helps prevent cerebral vasospasm
    - Persistent elevated blood pressure
        - Nitroprusside (Nipride) or Nicardipine (Cardene)

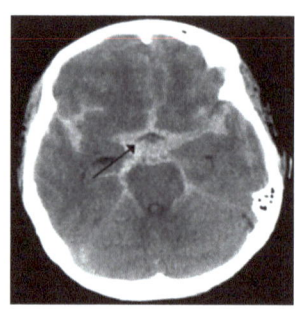

Diffuse Injuries
- Concussions
    - Mild (grade 1)
        - No loss of consciousness
        - May be accompanied by nausea, headache, confusion, and brief memory loss
        - Symptoms typically last less than an hour
    - Moderate (grade 2)
        - No loss or very brief loss of consciousness
        - Similar to grade 1 symptoms, but last between 30 minutes to a day
    - Severe (grade 3)
        - Unconsciousness followed by concussion symptoms
- Diffuse axonal injuries (DAI) (Coma)
    - Often due to rapid acceleration-deceleration forces

Cerebrovascular Accident (CVA)

- Disruption of blood flow to the brain resulting in a neurological deficit
    - Resolve within 24 hours: transient ischemic attack (TIA)
    - Persisting for more than 24 hours: stroke
- Assessment Tools
    - Cincinnati Prehospital Stroke Scale
    - Los Angeles Prehospital Stroke Scale
    - National Institute of Health Stroke Assessment

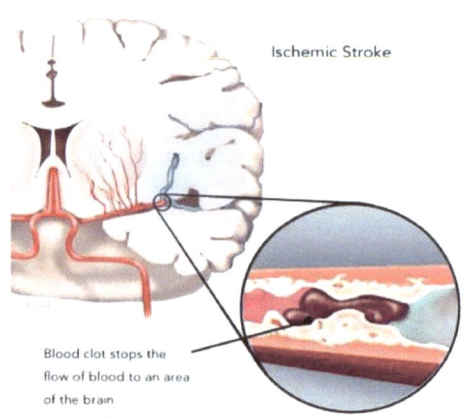

Stroke Management

If you suspect that your patient has new onset signs & symptoms of CVA, notify the cabin crew IMMEDIATELY! The medications discussed may have been part of your patient's care prior to transport.

- IV Thrombolytics at Stroke Hospital
- IA (intra-arterial) Thrombolytics at Stroke Hospital
- If hypertensive (>220/120mmHg)
    - Consider: Labetalol, Nitroprusside, Nicardipine (if available)
- Treat seizures with benzodiazepines/anticonvulsants per protocol
- *ELEVATE THE HEAD OF THE BED 30%*

Increased Intracranial Pressure (ICP)

Patients can have increased ICP for any number of reasons including trauma, tumors or masses, cerebral edema, etc. It is important to be able to recognize the symptoms of increasing ICP as it is a medical emergency and the cabin crew must be notified.

Clinical Features of Rising ICP
- Decreased level of consciousness
- Pupil reaction
- Posturing
    - Decorticate vs Decerebrate
- Changes in vital signs
- Cushing's Triad

Cushing's Triad
- Arterial Hypertension
    - Widened pulse pressures
- Bradycardia
- Respiratory Changes
    - Depend on the level of brainstem involved
    - Midbrain: Cheyne-Stokes respirations

Treatment of ICP
- *NOTIFY THE CABIN CREW OF THE MEDICAL EMERGENCY*
- Positioning of the patient, monitor for seizures and blood glucose levels
- Airway management and ventilation
- Consider osmotherapy, corticosteroids

Spinal Cord Injuries (SCI)

While your patient will have already been treated for their injury it is important to understand how their mobility can be affected, as well as longer term problems these patients can encounter.

Flexion-Extension Injuries
- Typically involve the cervical region
    - C3-4-5 keep the diaphragm alive
    - C5-C6 most susceptible
- Vertical Compression
- Rotation with Flexion

Complete vs. Incomplete Spinal Cord Injuries
- Complete
    - Complete disruption to anterior, middle and posterior tracks of the spinal cord
    - No sensory or motor function
    - C-Spine injury can result in quadriplegia
    - Thoracic injury can result in paraplegia
- Incomplete
    - Depending on the portion of the spinal cord involved, some motor, sensation, proprioception, etc. may be preserved

Spinal & Neurogenic Shock

Spinal Shock
- Temporary local neurologic condition after spinal trauma
    - Causes paralysis and absent reflexes
- Typically subsides within 24-72 hours

Neurogenic Shock
- Temporary loss of sympathetic nervous system outflow
- Classic presentation:
    - Hypotension
    - Bradycardia
    - Warm, Flushed, Dry below lesion
- Decreased Systemic Vascular Resistance (SVR) and low-normal heart rate (the tank is bigger)

Treatment of SCI
- Maintain ABCs
  - May have difficulty controlling secretions
- Treat neurogenic shock with vasoactive agents (if available)
  - The tank is bigger
- Treat bradycardia

Complications of SCI
- Autonomic dysreflexia (hyperreflexia)
  - Late complication
  - Commonly occurs with injuries above T6
- Bladder distension or irritation is responsible for 75-85% of the cases
  - Increases BP, HR, ICP
- Insert Foley and drain

Psychiatric Emergencies

Frequently repatriated commercially, these individuals may or may not have other clinical issues. Establishing a good rapport with your patient is key to a successful transport.

- Suicidal ideation – these patients have threatened to harm themselves
- Homicidal ideation – these patients have threated to harm others
- Schizophrenic – these patients are withdrawn from reality
- Bipolar disorder – these patients tend to have extremely high highs and extremely low lows
- Anxiety – these patients can be crippled by worry or fear

Management of Psychiatric Emergencies
- Safety
  - Recognizing when your and other passengers safety could be jeopardized
- Therapeutic communication
  - First line to de-escalation
- Non-pharmacologic restraints
  - Per your program's medical protocols, physical restraints may be utilized if needed.
- Pharmacologic restraints (IV or IM; oral is available)
  - Diphenhydramine (Benadryl) 25-50 mg
  - Droperidol (Inapsine) 2.5 mg
  - Haloperidol (Haldol) 5 mg
  - Lorazepam (Ativan) 2 mg

Sedatives
- Diphenhydramine: 25-50 mg by mouth or IM/IV every 4-6 hours as needed (max 300 mg/24 hours)
    - Contraindications: hypersensitivity, acute asthma, glaucoma
    - Common side effects: drowsiness, dizziness, dry mouth, blurred vision
- Droperidol: 2.5 mg IM or IV once. Additional 1.5 mg may be given with caution.
    - Contraindications: hypersensitivity, angle-closure glaucoma, CNS depression, severe liver or cardiac disease
    - Common side effects: hypotension, tachycardia, blurred vision, dry mouth, confusion, dizziness, extrapyramidal reactions
- Haloperidol (Haldol): 2.5 – 5 mg IM or IV every 1-8 hours PRN.
    - Contraindications: glaucoma, CNS depression, severe liver or cardiac disease
    - Common side effects: hypotension, blurred vision, dry mouth.
- Lorazepam (Ativan): generally, 2 mg IM or IV every 2 hours PRN
    - Contraindications: CNS depression, glaucoma, severe hypotension
    - Common side effects: dizziness, drowsiness, lethargy, mental depression

Respiratory Emergencies

While we cannot review every scenario you may encounter, some of the more common diagnoses are discussed.

Diagnostic Imaging

Use a systematic approach
- **A**irway Structures
    - Trachea, Carina, Bronchi
- **B**reathing Structures
    - Lungs, Pleura
- **C**ardiac
    - Heart size, borders
- **D**iaphragm
    - Costophrenic angles
- **E**verything else
    - Aorta, bones, tissue

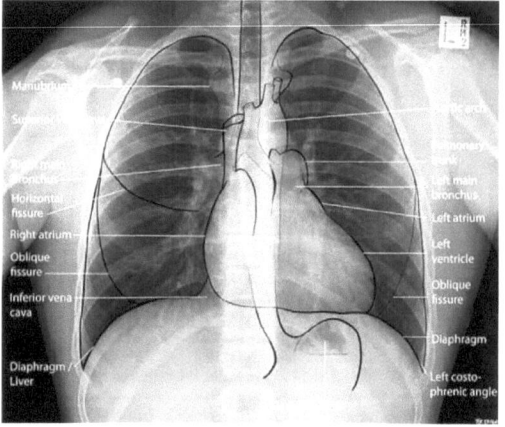

Respiratory System Review
- Anatomy
    - Air moves from the trachea, into the left and right bronchus. The bronchi further divide into smaller bronchi and finally into bronchioles. At the very end of the bronchial system are alveoli.

- Gas exchange
  - Gas exchange happens at the alveolar level where venules and arterioles meet at the capillary level.
- Alveoli
  - Millions of alveoli comprise lung tissue. When alveoli are not working properly, gas exchange is impaired.
- Atelectasis
  - Alveoli deflate for any number or reasons and are no longer capable of gas exchange.
  - May present with shortness of breath, fever, chest pain upon inhalation
  - Encourage the use of incentive spirometer and cough/deep breath, consider acetaminophen

Lobar Atelectasis

(https://www.youtube.com/watch?v=4oYBLkbDjhg)

Obstructive vs. Restrictive Lung Disease
- Obstructive Lung Disease
  - Hinders a person's ability to completely expel air from the lungs. The result is retained air in the lungs.
  - COPD, asthma, bronchiectasis, cystic fibrosis
- Restrictive Lung Disease:
  - People have a hard time fully expanding their lungs when they inhale. This can occur when tissue in the chest wall becomes stiffened, or due to weakened muscles or damaged nerves.
  - Interstitial lung disease, sarcoidosis, pulmonary fibrosis, neuromuscular disease

Your patient's diagnosis will allow you to anticipate their oxygen and ventilation needs in flight!

Asthma

Asthma exacerbation treatment
- Bronchodilators
- Steroids
- Anxiolytics for comfort if needed and available

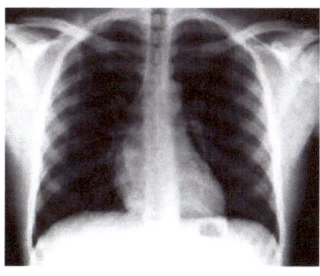

COPD

COPD exacerbation treatment
- Bronchodilators
- Steroids
- Anxiolytics for comfort if needed and available

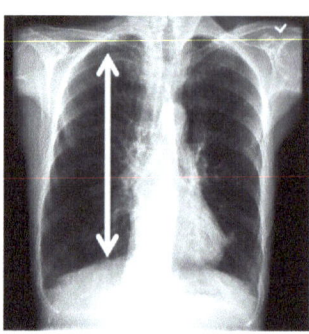

Pleural Effusion
- Fluid in the pleural space
- Will gravitate to most dependent area
- Treatment:
    - Evacuation or drainage
    - Pleural drain
    - Management of cause

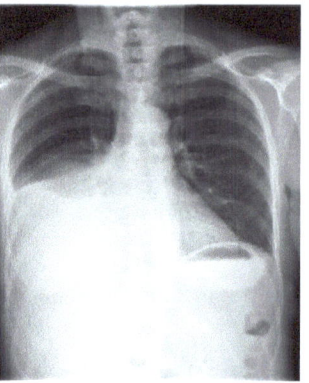

Pulmonary Embolism

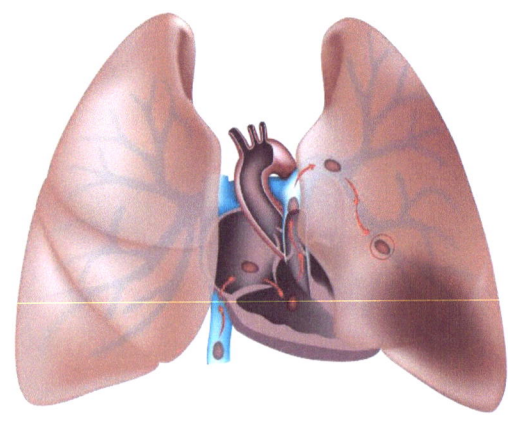

If you suspect that your patient has an acute pulmonary embolism in flight, rule out cardiac causes for chest pain and treat your patient symptomatically per your protocols.

Always evaluate the need to notify the cabin crew of the medical emergencies.

- Presentation
    - Your patient may have presented with chest pain, shortness of breath and/cough.
- Diagnosis
    - By the time you transfer your patient, they will have been diagnosed by CT or VQ scan and been started on a blood thinner to break up the clot.
- Treatment
    - You may need to assist the patient with self-injections of heparin or LMWH or with the administration of oral anticoagulants. Your patient may require supplemental oxygen and will probably tire easy.
- Further management
    - Ensure your patient has additional DVT prevention methods in place

Pneumonia
- Most often viral, sometimes bacterial
- Chest X-ray (CXR) shows pleural effusions, lobar consolidation
    - Right middle lobe pneumonia is the most common site of consolidation
    - Patchy infiltrates
- Pneumonia Treatment:
    - Bronchodilators, antibiotics, oxygen

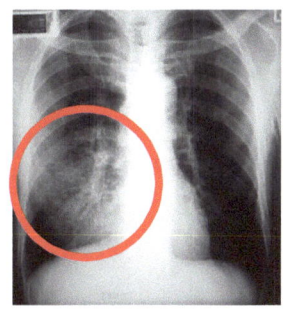

Basic Airway Management

During transport, should your patient deteriorate, they may require airway management. At this point, you should have already notified the cabin crew of the emergency. Based on your previous knowledge, experience and training, we will briefly discuss basic airway management.

Oropharyngeal Airways

Indications
- Unresponsive
- Lack of an intact gag
- Unable to protect airway
- Snoring respirations

Contraindications
- Responsive or semi-conscious patients
- Intact gag reflex
- Known or suspected palate injury

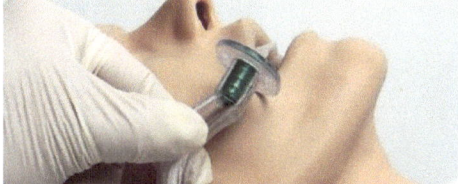

OPA Proper Sizing

Corner of the mouth to angle of the jaw

Nasopharyngeal Airway

Indications
- Unable to tolerate OPA
- Intact gag reflex
- Unresponsive or semi-conscious patients
- Unable to protect airway
- Snoring respirations

Contraindications
- Basilar skull fracture
- Facial trauma
- Disruption of the midface, nasopharynx or palate

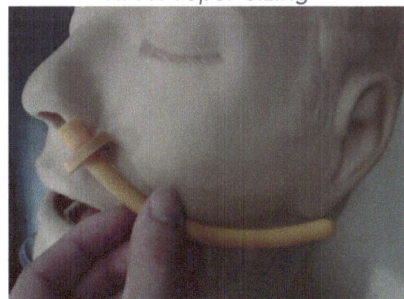

NPA Proper Sizing

Nare of insertion to the earlobe

Bag Mask Ventilation
- Place thumb and index finger of one hand over the mask in the shape of a "C" and push down
- Place the other three fingers under the mandible and lift the mandible up (jaw thrust) forming an "E"
- Only enough of a bag squeeze for adequate chest rise.
- 12 to 20 breaths per minute, or per your protocols

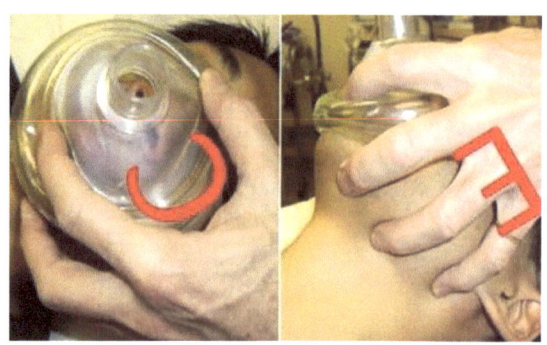

Supraglottic Devices

These devices may be a part of your program's scope of practice. Additional training per their policies should be available.

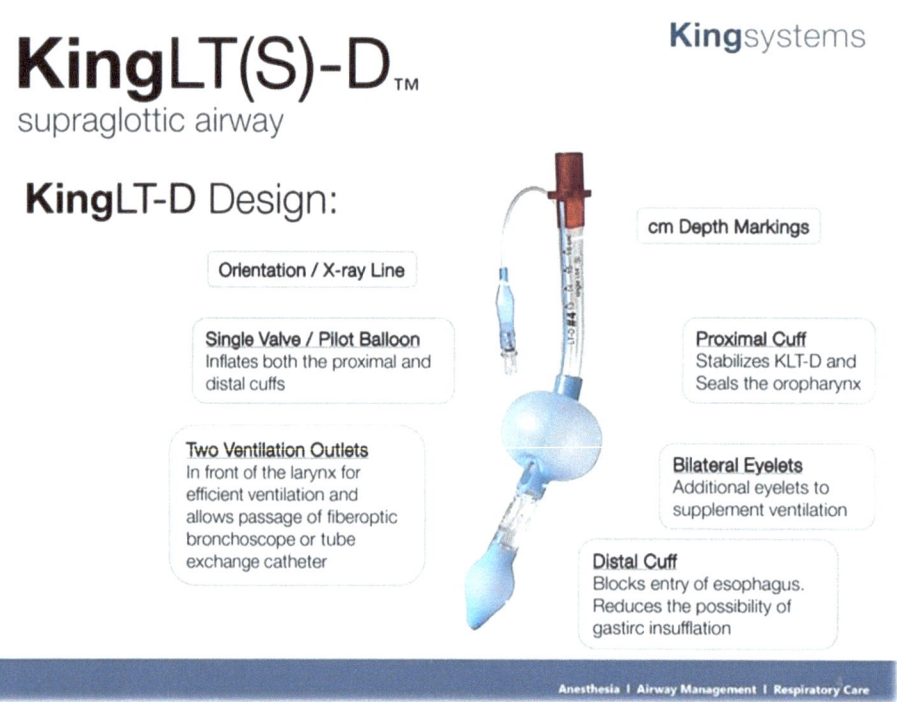

- Ability to be placed without direct visualization
- Provides rapid airway intervention in the field
- Provides little protection against aspiration
- Risk of mucosal damage and blood flow reduction if the wrong size is utilized or balloon is overinflated

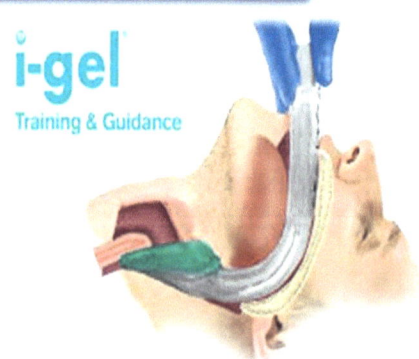

Facial Trauma & Airway Management

Any instability of the bones of the face can impede your ability to manage their airway, if needed. Maxillofacial trauma can cause airway obstruction including loose teeth, soft tissue swelling, etc.

Orbital Fractures
- Potentially lead to the instability of the maxilla

Le Forte Fractures
- Le Forte I: Horizontal across the maxilla, maxilla and maxillary teeth are moveable
- Le Forte II: Bridge of nose and around the mouth, usually from a downward blow to the nose
- Le Forte III: Transverse Fracture, aka "Craniofacial Dissociation"
- Treatment could involve surgical repair, including but not limited to jaw wiring.

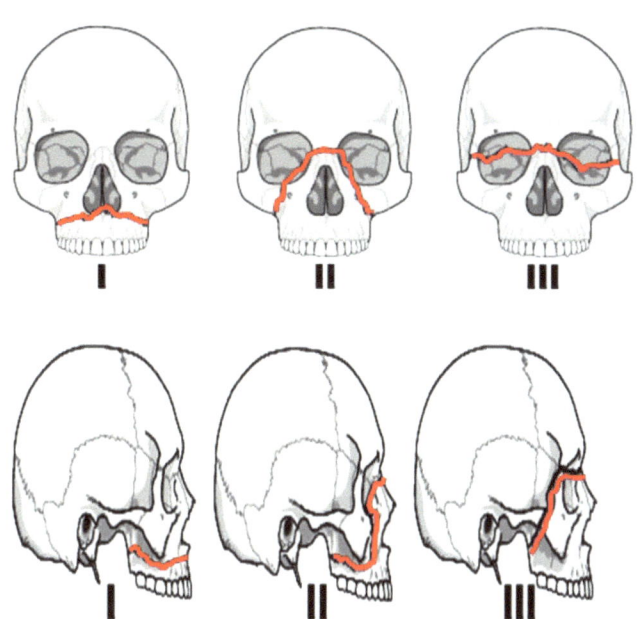

Cardiac Emergencies

Based on your prior knowledge, a brief review of common cardiac diagnoses that are common reasons for commercial repatriation. Any disruption in the electrical or mechanical systems can lead to cardiac arrhythmias or failure.

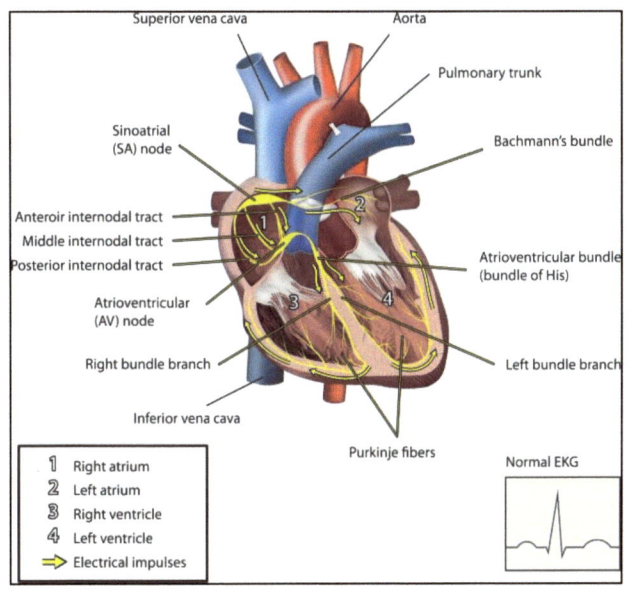
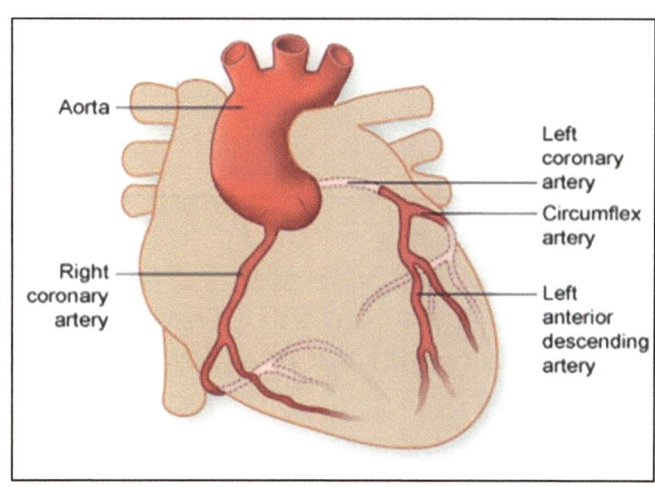

Acute Coronary Syndrome
- Angina- Non-occlusive decrease in flow
    - Non-specific ECG Changes
    - Normal Enzymes
    - Stable vs. Unstable vs. Variant (Prinzmetal)
- STEMI- Occlusive thrombus
    - Specific ECG Changes
    - Elevated enzymes
- NSTEMI- non-occlusive thrombus
    - Non-specific ECG Changes
    - Elevated enzymes

Acute Myocardial Infarction Treatment
- Oxygen per protocol and patient need to keep SpO_2 >92%
- Reduce preload/pain relief
    - Morphine not routinely used, unless other pain management options are not available
- Coronary dilation
- Reduce HR/O_2 demand (Beta Blockers/CCBs)
- Clot Prevention (ASA, clopidogrel [Plavix] or ticagrelor [Brillinta])
- Reperfusion (Chemical or Surgical)
- MONA or FONA used as a mnemonic to remember initial treatment

Congestive Heart Failure (CHF)

CHF is caused by the cardiac pump's failure to adequately circulate blood. This causes a backup, terminating in the lungs. The patient with severe and decompensated CHF is most likely not fit to fly. [9]

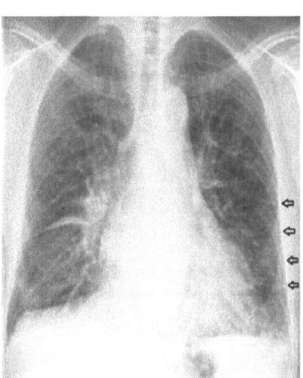

- Patient presents with progressive dyspnea, coughing up frothy sputum, etc.
- Most common cause of right heart failure is left heart failure
- Can happen suddenly

CHF Treatment
- Noninvasive positive pressure ventilation
- Nitroglycerine
- Diuretic therapy to decrease preload
- Angiotensin Converting Enzyme Inhibitors (ACE Inhibitors) to prevent ventricular remodeling

Cardiac Medications
- Aspirin: 80-325 mg once daily. If acute MI is suspected, 160 mg immediately.
  - Contraindications: bleeding disorders
  - Common side effects: epigastric pain, rash, GI bleeding
- Furosemide (Lasix): 40 mg IV or IM every 12 hours.
  - Contraindications: anuria
  - Common side effects: dizziness, hypotension, dehydration, dry mouth, hypokalemia
- Nitroglycerin: spray – 1-2 sprays every 5 minutes, max 3 doses. Sublingual – 0.3-0.6 mg every 5 minutes, max 3 doses. Transdermal (paste) – 1-2" every 6-8 hours.
  - Contraindications: hypersensitivity, hypotension
  - Common side effects: headache, dizziness, hypotension, tachycardia

Gastrointestinal Disorders

This brief review is meant to build on your experience and knowledge of GI disorders. Applying the gas laws and flight physiology will guide you in your patient care.

Gastrointestinal Bleeding

You patient may have received blood transfusions prior to commercial transfer.

- Upper: Gastritis, NSAID use, alcohol, ulcers
  - Treated via Esophagogastroduodenoscopy with epi injections, banding, etc.
    - Esophagus
    - Stomach
    - Duodenum
- Lower: diverticulitis, hernias, adhesions, inflammatory bowel diseases, cancer
  - Treated during a colonoscopy with epi injections, banding, etc.
  - Small intestines: Difficult to stop bleeding without surgical intervention.
  - Large intestines

Bowel Obstructions

Small bowel obstructions can be caused by scarring from prior surgeries, hernia or cancer. They can be managed conservatively with NG tube placement for decompression. Alternatively, they may require surgery.

Large bowel obstructions can be caused by a tumor/cancer, volvulus (twisting of the bowels), strictures/scarring or an Intussusception where a part of the bowel slides into another part. These types often require surgery.

Prior to commercial transfer, your patient must be passing flatus and should be having regular bowel movements. An unresolved bowel obstruction with trapped gas is a contraindication to commercial transport!

Ostomies require close monitoring for gaseous expansion

Nausea/Vomiting/Diarrhea

Common during overseas travel and can be caused by food and drink. Air sickness occurs as well. These issues may not be related to any diagnosis or side effect.

Treat your patient according to your protocol for their comfort.

GI Medications
- Antacids: 1-2 chews every 4 hours as needed
    - Contraindications: severe abdominal pain of unknown origin, renal failure
    - Common side effects: constipation or diarrhea (depending on type given)
- Loperamide (Imodium): 4 mg by mouth after 1st loose stool, followed by 2 mg after each subsequent loose stool (max 8 mg/day).
    - Contraindications: abdominal pain of unknown origin.
    - Common side effects: constipation, drowsiness, dizziness, dry mouth
- Meclizine (Dramamine): 25 mg by mouth every 6 hours as needed
    - Contraindications:, pregnancy, glaucoma
    - Common side effects: drowsiness, blurred vision, dry mouth
- Ondansetron (Zofran): 4 mg ODT or IM/IV every 6 hours as needed.
    - Contraindications: none significant
    - Common side effects: headache, dizziness, drowsiness, diarrhea, constipation, dry mouth

Metabolic & Endocrine Disorders

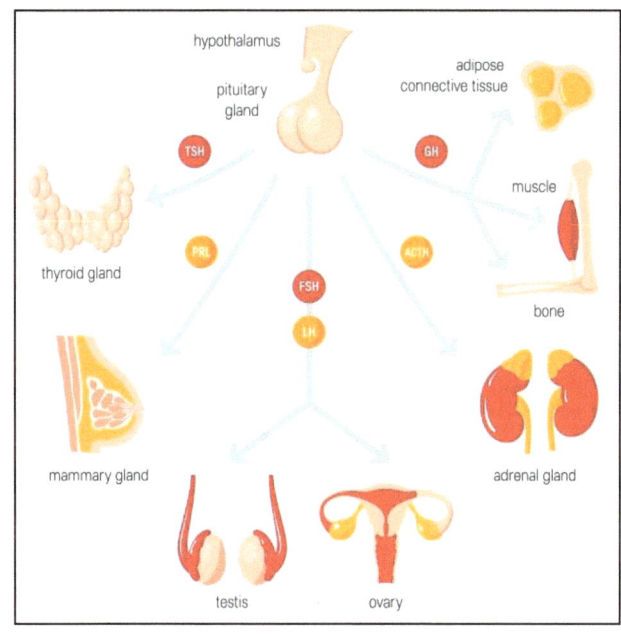

Diabetes
- Type 1
- Type 2 (90% of all Diabetic patients)
- Gestational

You may have to assist your patient with the administration of insulin or oral antihyperglycemic agents.

Should your patient become HYPOglycemic and they can manage their airway/secretions, administer oral glucose, juice, cola, etc. Make sure they receive an extra meal and continue to monitor their blood glucose.

- Oral glucose: 10-20 grams by mouth. May repeat every 10-20 minutes if needed.

Diabetic Ketoacidosis (DKA)
- Most common in Type I diabetic teens/children
    - Life threatening
- Elevated glucose (>350mg/dL)
    - Rarely exceeds 800 mg/dL
- Ketones
- Metabolic Acidosis
- Respiratory Alkalosis due to Kussmaul respirations

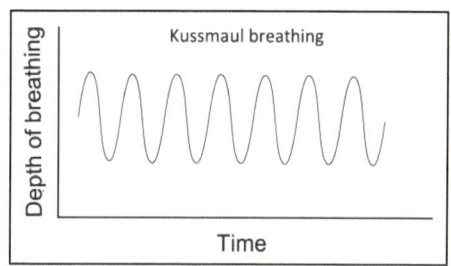

Hyperglycemic Hyperosmolar Non-Ketosis (HHNK)
- May also be referred to as HHS or HHNS
- Common with Type II Diabetes
- Extremely elevated glucose (>600mg/dL)
    - Sometimes >1000mg/dL
- Polydipsia, Polyuria, Polyphagia
- Normal ketones (non-ketotic)
    - No significant acid/base disturbance

If your patient was treated for severe blood glucose disturbances, their blood chemistries will have been corrected prior to transport. Their treatment may have included insulin administration, fluid resuscitation and potassium correction.

Pituitary Disorders

Diabetes Insipidus (DI) vs. Syndrome of Inappropriate Antidiuretic Hormone (SIADH)

Diabetes Insipidus
- High urine output, low urine osmolarity
- Requires copious amounts of fluids
- Requires vasopressin/desmopressin (DDAVP) to retain fluids.
- Neurogenic vs nephrogenic causes

SIADH
- Pituitary gland releases excessive amounts of ADH
- Causes:
  - Disease
  - TCA
  - Narcotics
  - Oral hypoglycemic agents
- Dilutional hyponatremia is the problem

Hypothyroidism

- Very common, treated with Levothyroxine
- Patient presents with fatigue, cold intolerance, puffy eyelids, sparse hair, possible goiter
- Can progress to Myxedema Coma
  - Cold exposure
  - Infection
  - Trauma
  - Stroke
  - Drugs

Hyperthyroidism

- Excessive levels can lead to thyroid storm/thyrotoxicosis/Graves Disease
- Increased metabolism
- Treated with beta blockers and antithyroid drugs

Adrenal Insufficiency

Addison's Disease
- Autoimmune
- Can be caused by abrupt changes in steroid use
- Presents with altered mental status, shock, severe pain in lower extremities, severe vomiting and diarrhea
- Treatment includes steroids and weaning them to zero.

Hypercortisolism

Cushing's Syndrome
- Presents with 'buffalo hump,' moon face, thin arms/legs, purple striae on abdomen
- Causes: excessive use of corticosteroids, tumors
- Usually resolves when corticosteroids are stopped or tumor is removed

Environmental & Toxicology Emergencies

Thermoregulatory Issues
Your patient will have been treated and stabilized prior to commercial transport.

Heat
- Heat Cramps
  - Profuse sweating, hyponatremia
- Heat exhaustion
  - Water depleted
  - Sodium depleted
- Heat stroke
  - Altered Mental status
- Electrolyte imbalances

Cold
- Frostbite
- Hypothermia
  - Mild (90°-95° F or 32.2°-35° C)
  - Severe (below 90° F or 32.2° C)
  - Electrolyte Imbalances

Envenomation
Snake bites can cause coagulopathy and scorpions can cause a great deal of pain and occasional neuromuscular dysfunction.

Acetaminophen Overdose

- Most commonly ingested drug resulting in overdose
- Toxic signs and symptoms delayed, causes severe liver damage

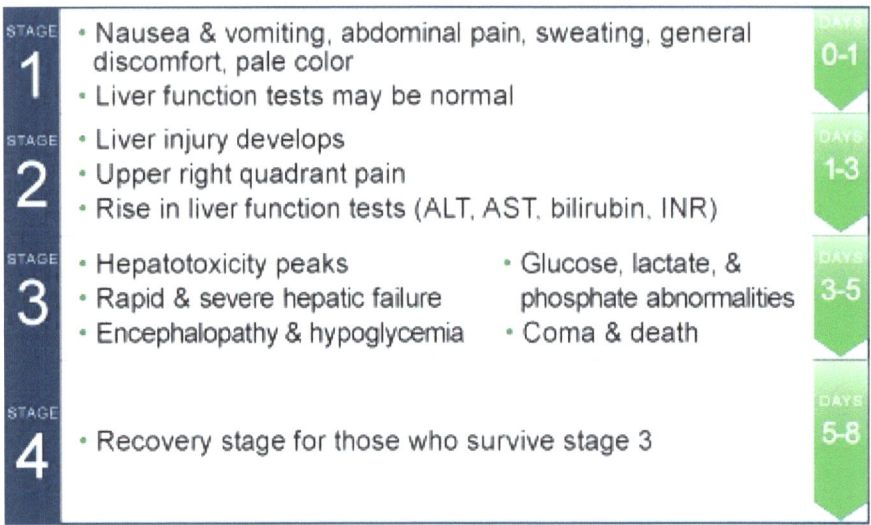

STAGE 1 (Days 0-1)
- Nausea & vomiting, abdominal pain, sweating, general discomfort, pale color
- Liver function tests may be normal

STAGE 2 (Days 1-3)
- Liver injury develops
- Upper right quadrant pain
- Rise in liver function tests (ALT, AST, bilirubin, INR)

STAGE 3 (Days 3-5)
- Hepatotoxicity peaks
- Rapid & severe hepatic failure
- Encephalopathy & hypoglycemia
- Glucose, lactate, & phosphate abnormalities
- Coma & death

STAGE 4 (Days 5-8)
- Recovery stage for those who survive stage 3

Anticholinergic Poisoning

Drugs like
- Atropine
- Scopolamine (motion sickness)
- Chlorpheniramine (Deconamine)
- Hydroxyzine (Atarax)
- Dimenhydrinate (Dramamine)
- Diphenhydramine (Benadryl)
- Meclizine (Antivert)
- Promethazine (Phenergan)
- Cyclic antidepressants (TCAs)

Anticholinergic Toxidrome
- Mad as a hatter — Altered mental status
- Blind as a bat — Mydriasis
- Red as a beet — Flushed skin
- Hot as a hare — Dry skin (anhydrosis)
- Dry as a bone — Dry mucous membranes

Diving Injuries
- All divers are subject to pressure effects
- Nitrogen dissolves into fatty tissues
    - Displaces O_2 in the brain
    - Nitrogen Narcosis
- Expands during ascent
    - Bends
    - Boyle's Law
- As a general rule, divers should avoid flying for 24-48 hours after dive completion

> Was your patient on holiday and diving?

Decompression Sickness
- Type I
    - Painful, mottled skin, pruritic (itching)
- Type II
    - Neurologic signs and symptoms, hypovolemic shock

Dive-Associated Barotrauma
- Ascent or descent
- Pulmonary Overpressurization Syndrome (POPS)
    - "Breath Holding"
    - Pneumothorax
    - Subcutaneous or mediastinal emphysema
- Greatest pressure changes occur 4 feet below the surface

Arterial Gas Embolism
- Patient presents with stroke-like symptoms
- May also have a cough and epistaxis nosebleed
- AGE requires immediate hyperbaric treatment

Any patient to be transported commercially must have all dive-related and barotrauma-related injuries resolved due to Boyle's Law.

Altitude Illness
- Hypoxia is the main culprit in altitude sickness
    - Low atmospheric pressures
- Pre-existing medical conditions
    - Extremes of age
    - Sedentary lifestyles
    - Poor overall health

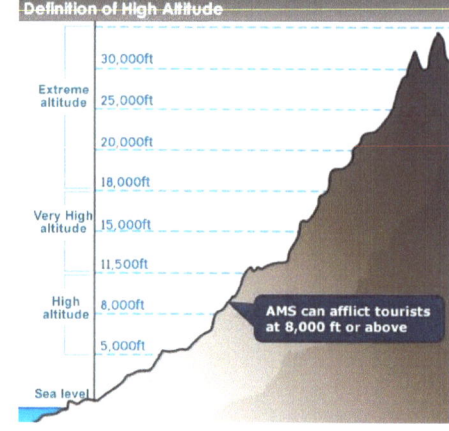

Acute Mountain Sickness
- Rapid Ascent
    - Symptoms begin within 24 hours
- Descend in altitude
- Lake Louise Criteria
    - Recent gain in altitude >8200 feet (>2500 m)
    - Headache
    - Symptomatic
        - GI symptoms, dizziness fatigue or weakness, difficulty sleeping

High-Altitude Pulmonary Edema (HAPE)

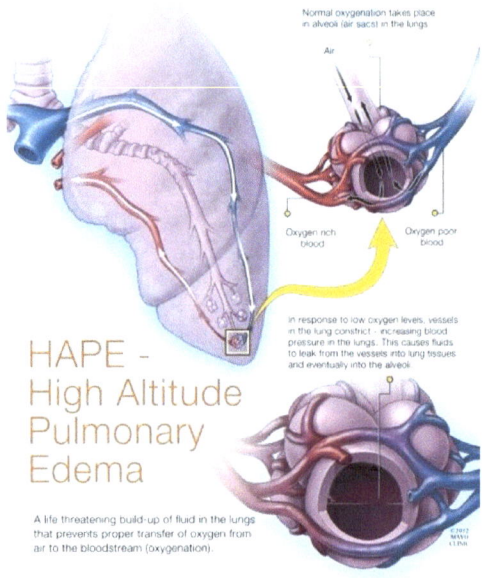

- Onset occurs 2-4 days after rapid ascent > 10,000 ft.
- Symptoms:
    - Rales
    - Tachycardia
    - Tachypnea
    - Dyspnea at rest
    - Fever
    - Non-productive cough
    - May have pink frothy sputum
- Treatment:
    - DESCENT
    - Supplemental O_2
    - CPAP may be necessary in the acute phase

Image: www.mayoclinic.org

High-Altitude Cerebral Edema (HACE)

- Considered a life-threatening emergency
    - Mental status changes and/or ataxia after rapid ascent, often >12,000 ft. MSL
    - Typically after 5 days at sustained high altitudes
    - Occurs the latest of all altitude injuries
    - Visual changes
    - Paresthesia
    - Mental status changes
    - Coma
- Treatment
    - Descend
    - Dexamethasone

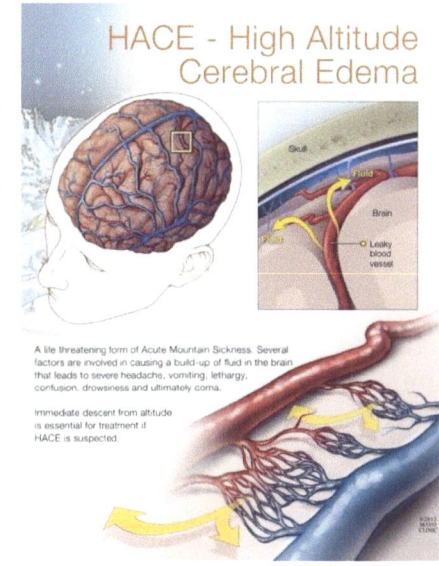

Image: www.mayoclinic.org

Trauma Patient Management

Your patient may have been involved in a traumatic accident. We will discuss common mechanisms of trauma. Depending on your patient's mechanism of injury (motor vehicle crash, motorcycle crash, fall, gunshot, etc.) they may have a variety of injuries. While your patient has been stabilized and injuries (possibly) surgically repaired, it is important to understand what they have been through.

Types of Trauma

- Blunt: assault, motor vehicle crash, fall, etc.
    - Deceleration
    - Shearing, rupture of body organs
- Penetrating
    - Stab wounds
    - Gunshot wounds
        - High velocity weapons fire projectiles >2000

Hypovolemic Shock

- Too little circulating blood within the vascular system
    - HR increases
    - SVR increases
    - CO drops
- Cold extremities and worsening mental status
- Early fluid resuscitation and blood products

Falls
- Most common: hip fracture
- Pelvic fracture
- Axial loading on the spine causes compression fractures
- Bilateral wrist fractures (bracing while falling)

Abdominal Trauma

The abdominal cavity is home to many vital organs in a large space without much protection. Injury can lead to severe blood loss without significant outward signs.

Splenic Rupture
- Most commonly injured solid organ in blunt trauma
- Often associated with MVC's
- Potentially asymptomatic
- Abdominal tenderness or referred pain
  - Positive Kehr's sign
- Surgical intervention is often required

Liver
- Most commonly injured solid organ in penetrating trauma
  - Extremely vascular
- Risk of shearing in sudden deceleration

Large & Small intestine
- Most commonly injured *hollow* organ from penetrating trauma
- Significant risk for sepsis due to bacteria

Thoracic Trauma

Pneumothorax
- Accumulation of air in the thoracic cavity, blunt or penetrating trauma
- Spontaneous pneumo is from rupture of blebs
- Open pneumothorax
  - Sucking chest wound
- Must be resolved or chest drain in place prior to transport

Rib Fracture
- Can be diagnosed clinically based on history and presentation
- Ribs 1-3
    - Associated with head, neck, spinal cord injuries
- Ribs 10-12
    - Associated with liver and spleen injuries
- Treat with analgesics
- Ensure the patient takes deep breaths
    - Prevents atelectasis
    - Decreases risk for pneumonia

Burn Management

General burn considerations
- Pain management
    - May require more than anticipated
- Dressings
    - Helps prevent infection. Use sterile gloves when required.
- Risk of infection
    - Administer antibiotics as ordered
- Nutrition
    - Assist your patient to follow their prescribed diet
- Fluid balance
    - Encourage PO and electrolyte intake

Classification of Thermal Burns
- 1st Degree or Superficial: Sunburns
- 2nd Degree or Partial thickness: Blisters
- 3rd Degree or Full thickness: Completely destroyed tissue

Electrical Burn Considerations
- Voltage
- Resistance
    - Degree of hindrance to flow of electricity
- Type of pathway and current
    - Nerves, blood vessels and muscles have low resistance and transmit easily.
    - Fat and tendons are the most resistant and do not conduct electricity easily.

Your patient may have extensive internal injuries, including but not limited to renal failure, most likely rhabdomyolysis.

Acid & Alkali Burns

While they both have different mechanisms of burn, understand that soft tissue will most likely be involved.

Again, these patients will most likely need more pain medications than other patients.

Some chemical burns can be to the face– your patient may be disfigured and also have emotional needs as well.

Post-Surgical Patients
- Pain Management
    - Assist your patient as needed. Follow your protocols if narcotic pain medication is provided by your program
- Mobility
    - Arm vs. leg vs. back vs. abdomen
    - May be limited by pain
- Infection
    - Continue antibiotics
- Dressings
    - Change per order and as needed
- Anemia & oxygenation
    - Generally speaking, your patient's Hgb should be >8.0 for travel
    - Provide oxygen as needed and available

External Fixators
- External hardware that secures fractured bones
- Heavy
- Impaired movement/mobility
    - A wrist ex-fix is easier to manage than a lower leg ex-fix.
- Patient comfort
    - Talk to the cabin crew regarding patient positioning during taxi/takeoff/landing.

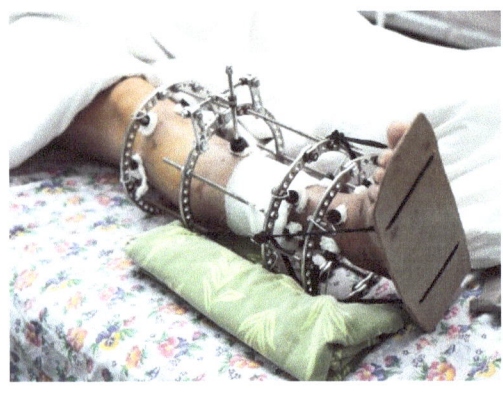
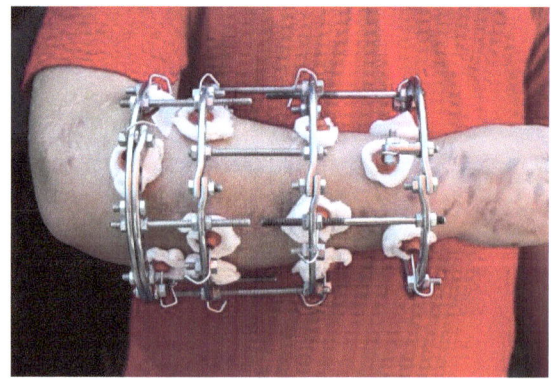

Drains

- Drains can be anywhere in your patient's body.
- Most often times, seen in the abdomen or chest.
- There are several types of drains you may encounter for commercial transport::
    - Pigtail, compression, chest tube.
- Keep in mind that you may need to empty it during travel.
- A properly functioning drain is safe for commercial travel as it will gather any air collections.
- *Note: drains with a valve or 3-way stop may be "burped" during transport*
- Monitor drain output as well as the dressing that may need to be changed.
- Any patient complaints or changes need to be investigated as the drain may require irrigation.

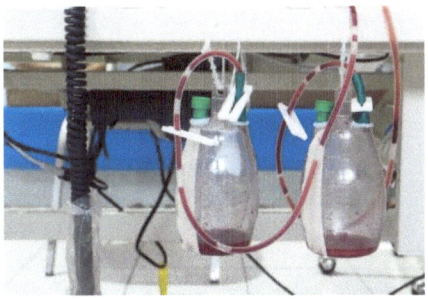
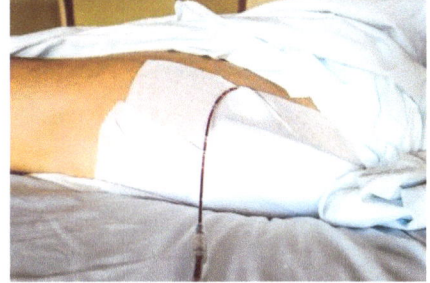
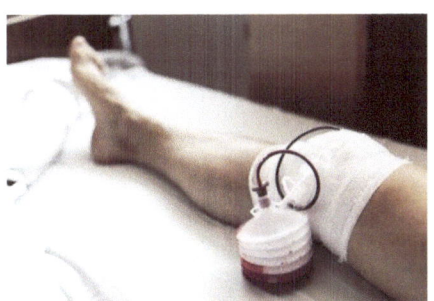
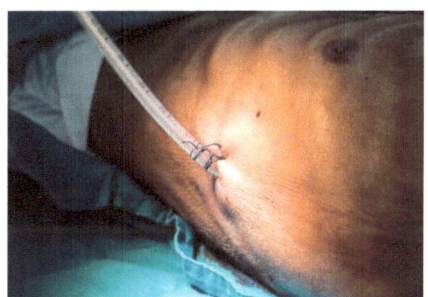

Pain Management
- Acetaminophen (Tylenol): 325 mg - 650 mg by mouth every 4-6 hours as needed (max 4 grams/24 hours)
    - Contraindications: hypersensitivity, severe hepatic disease
    - Common side effects: rash
- Ibuprofen (Motrin): 400 mg by mouth every 4-6 hours as needed (max 3.6 grams/24 hours)
    - Contraindications: hypersensitivity, active GI bleed or ulcer disease
    - Common side effects: headache, dizziness, GI upset
- Ketorolac (Toradol): 10-20 mg by mouth every 4-6 hours (max 40 mg/day). 30 mg IM or IV every 6 hours (max 120 mg/24 hours).
    - Contraindications: hypersensitivity, severe cardiovascular disease, severe renal disease
    - Common side effects: drowsiness, dizziness, increased bleeding time, dyspnea

Miscellaneous Basic Pharmacology

Medications for Allergic Reactions
- Epinephrine Auto Injector: 0.3 mg IM every 15-30 minutes as needed
    - Contraindicated in: cardiac arrythmias
    - Common side effects: hypertension, restlessness, nervousness, tachycardia
- Diphenhydramine: 25-50 mg by mouth or IM/IV every 4-6 hours as needed (max 300 mg/24 hours)
    - Contraindicated in: hypersensitivity, acute asthma, glaucoma
    - Common side effects: drowsiness, dizziness, dry mouth, blurred vision

Conclusion

The most vital thing to remember is to notify the cabin crew of any deterioration of your patient that is beyond your ability to manage.

Utilizing your prior knowledge and experience, this brief overview of anatomy, physiology and pathophysiology combined with flight physiology prepares you to succeed.

Your patient has been stabilized to the point of being declared FTF commercially.

Understanding what your patient has been through as part of their clinical course allows you understand how to take amazing care of your patients during commercial transport.

Keeping in mind that every agency's medical protocols are different and carries different medications (including medications potentially not available in other countries), the brief pharmacology overview helps you understand how to treat certain patient complaints.

ALS & CRITICAL CARE IN THE COMMERCIAL ENVIRONMENT 5

Equipment

 Depending on the equipment your program uses, the following may be a single unit or each entity may be separate. Ensure *equipment redundancy in the event of equipment or power failure.*

- Cardiac Monitor
    - Cardiac monitoring/EKG
    - Transcutaneous pacing
    - Synchronized cardioversion
    - Defibrillation
    - NIBP & IBP
    - SPO_2/$EtCO_2$ monitoring
- Intravenous Pump
    - Number of channels
    - Programmable for titration
    - Syringe driver
    - Medication and/or fluid bags
- Ventilators
    - Different brands
- Suction
    - Battery powered, 300 mmHG power
- Encapsulated ICU
    - Available on certain airlines and routes
    - Fully equipped and stocked with medication, equipment, etc.
        - Monitor
        - Defibrillator
        - iSTAT
        - Ventilator
        - IV pumps
        - Etc.
    - Physician and nurse provided
        - On occasion, you may be providing care with the physician

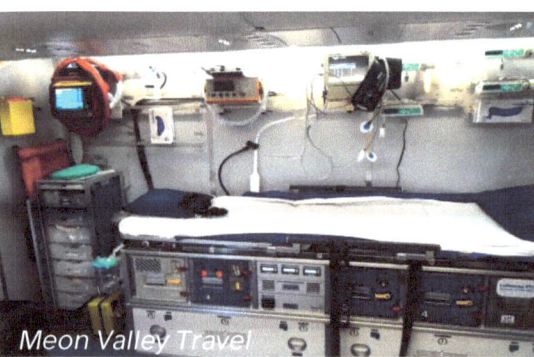
Meon Valley Travel

Critical Care Concepts

Based on your prior knowledge, experience and training, we will go over concepts in the management of critical care patients.

Neuro Patients

Normal Cranial Perfusion Values
- **Mean Arterial Pressure: 70-110 mmHg**
- **Intracranial Pressure: 0-15 cm H_2O**
    - 20mmHg has high mortality
- **Cerebral Perfusion Pressure: 70-90 mmHg**
    - Minimum pressure required to perfuse the brain. Must not fall below 70

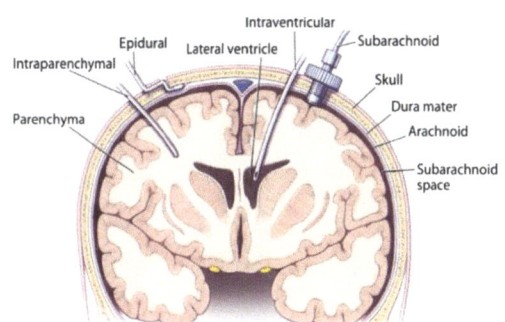

Mean Arterial Pressure (MAP) Formula
DBP + 1/3 Pulse Pressure (SBP-DBP)

-or-

$$\frac{(2 \times DBP) + SBP}{3}$$

Cerebral Perfusion Pressure (CPP) Formula
MAP – ICP (70 – 90 mmHg)

ICP Waveform

Goal of monitoring is to improve the ability to maintain adequate CPP and oxygenation. Transducer is placed at the Foramen of Monro.

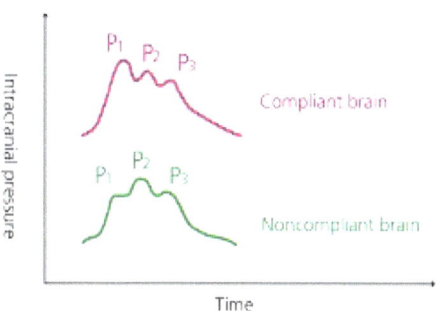

- Early detection of intracranial hypertension (ICP >15)
- Waveform has 3 parts:
    - P_1: Percussion wave – Arterial pulsation
    - P_2: Tidal wave – intracranial compliance
    - P_3: Dicrotic wave – venous
        - P_2 - P_3 Aortic valve Closing

> Hypoxia and Hypercapnia cause cerebral blood vessels to dilate, increasing blood flow and volume, further escalating ICP.

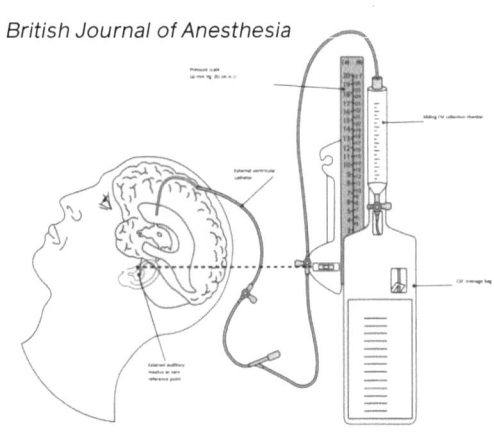
British Journal of Anesthesia

External Ventricular Drains (CSF)

- Used for the management of hydrocephalus
- Leveled at the Foramen of Monro
  - Too low or high can case over/under drainage
- Can monitor ICP (not a digital waveform)
- Allows for sampling of CSF
- CO_2 and electrolyte monitoring
  - Na 140-45

Hypertensive Abnormalities

Hypertensive Urgency
- Condition where a patient has extremely elevated blood pressure with no signs or symptoms of end organ damage
- Blood pressure should be lowered slowly
- Not an emergency

Hypertensive Crisis/Emergency
- Elevated blood pressure plus symptoms of end organ damage
- Headache, nausea/vomiting, visual changes
- Creatinine/RBCs in urine due to increased arterial pressure
- Treatment:
  - Lower BP no more than **25%** per hour, and no lower than patients' "normal" pressure
  - Labetalol, Nitroprusside, Nicardipine

Respiratory Patients

Acute Respiratory Distress Syndrome (ARDS)

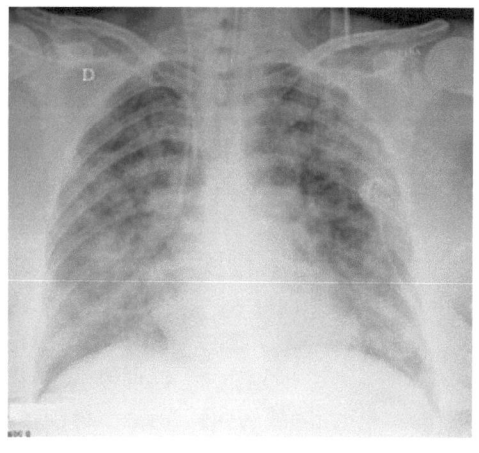

ARDS is the most severe form of Acute Lung Injury (ALI), a form of diffuse alveolar injury. It is characterized by increased permeability of the alveolar-capillary barrier, leading to an influx of fluid into the alveolar space. This results in hypoxemia and pulmonary hypertension, which further contributes to the V/Q mismatch.

- Caused by:
    - Pancreatitis
    - Sepsis
    - Trauma
    - Aspiration Pneumonia
- Chest X-ray shows:
    - "Ground glass appearance"
    - "Patchy infiltrates"
    - "Bilateral diffuse infiltrates"
- Swan-Ganz
    - Patient has a high PAWP (18-20 mmHg)
    - This pressure is higher than normal because the right heart is pumping against increased resistance in the lung vasculature

ARDS Treatment:
- Focus on oxygenation with:
    - ↑PEEP (>10 cm H_2O) & ↑ FiO_2
    - Low tidal volumes (4cc/kg)
    - Increase Rate (F)
        - Ensure adequate minute volume
- Follow ARDSnet Guidelines

Advanced Airway Management

Commercial Transport Specific Pearls
- Interfacility transfer
    - On a basic level, your patient is IN a facility
    - This transfer could have taken days to weeks to plan
    - Airway may have already been managed prior to your arrival
- Capabilities within the hospital
    - Is the environment at the discharging facility more conducive to manage the patient's airway?
- Limited working environment on the aircraft
    - Managing an airway on a stretcher or routine seat can be challenging
    - Airway management competence is vital
- Forward thinking
    - What are your patient's anticipated airway management needs?
    - Manage them at the discharging hospital PRIOR to boarding the aircraft

Airway Assessment

Indications for Airway Management
- Protection of the airway
    - Patient cannot manage secretions, GCS < 8
- Positive pressure
    - Insufficient ventilatory effort
- Partial pressure of oxygen
    - Need for higher FiO_2 or mean airway pressures
- Pulmonary toilet
    - Remove blood, secretions, infections
- Patient progression
    - *Likely to develop need*

> ***Severe acidosis***
> ***Hypercarbia***
> ***Hypoxia***

Difficult Intubation Predictors
- LEMON
- HEAVEN

LEMON
Look externally
Evaluate 3-3-2
Mallampati I-IV
Obstructions
Neck Mobility

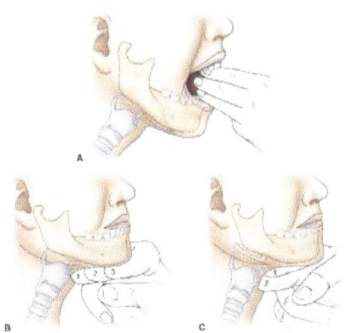

Image: Walls Manual of Emergency Management

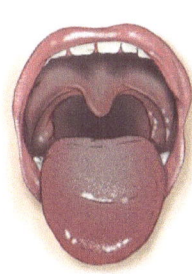
Class I
Entire posterior pharynx is fully exposed

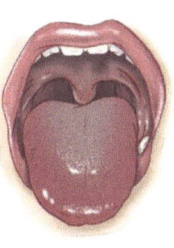
Class II
Posterior pharynx is partially exposed

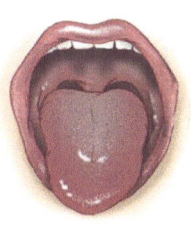
Class III
Posterior pharynx cannot be seen; base of the uvula is exposed

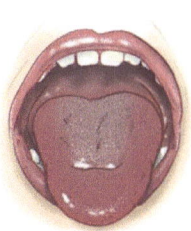
Class IV
No posterior pharyngeal structures can be seen

HEAVEN
Hypoxemia
    O_2 saturation less than 93% at the time of initial laryngoscopy
Extremes of size
    Patient less than or equal to 8 years of age or clinical obesity
Anatomic challenges
    Trauma, mass, swelling, foreign body, or other structural abnormality limiting view
Vomit/blood/fluid
    Clinically significant fluid in the pharynx or hypopharynx
Exsanguination/anemia
    Suspected anemia that could potentially accelerate the rate of decompensation during RSI apneic period
Neck mobility issues

Equipment & Patient Positioning

Ramping
- Ear to sternal notch positioning
- Improved upper airway patency
- Decreased work of breathing
- Prolonged safe apnea period

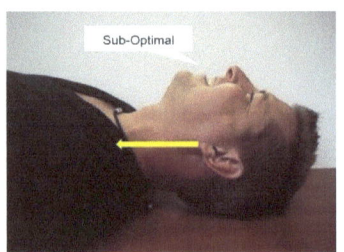 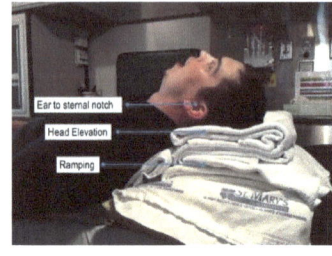

Note: Patients left in the supine position during intubation or transport causes a potential decrease in functional reserve capacity (FRC), tidal volume (Vt), and preload which can further potentiate injury or illness

Image: Walls Manual of Emergency Management

Intubation Equipment

Macintosh Blade
- Lifts the epiglottis via the vallecula

Miller Blade
- Direct displacement of the epiglottis
- Preferred method for neonates, infants, and young children

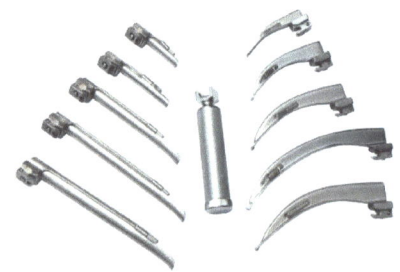

Video Laryngoscope
- Form of indirect laryngoscopy where the clinician views the larynx on a video screen
- Aids in visualization and difficult airways
- May have the capability to record the entire procedure

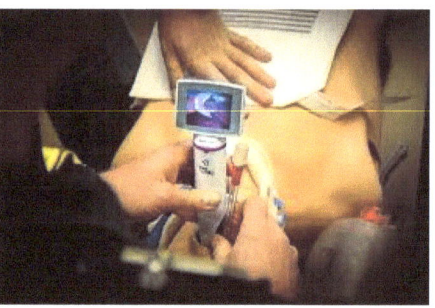

Bougie/Introducer   Adult: 15 Fr [ETT >6.0]   Pediatric: 10 Fr [ETT >4.0]
- Assists in intubation
- Surgical airway
- Confirmation of endotracheal tube position
- Endotracheal tube exchange
- Tracheal intubation via direct or video laryngoscopy, especially in difficult airways or during CPR

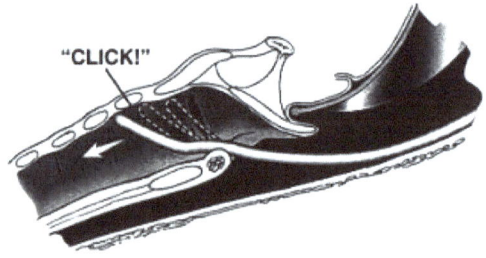

Placement Confirmation

Chest X-Ray
Gold standard of placement (depth) confirmation
- Distal tip of ETT should be:
    - 4-5 cm above the carina
    - At the level of the T3-T4 vertebrae
    - Can quickly be confirmed by visualizing Murphy's eye where the clavicles meet
- Visualization and waveform capnography

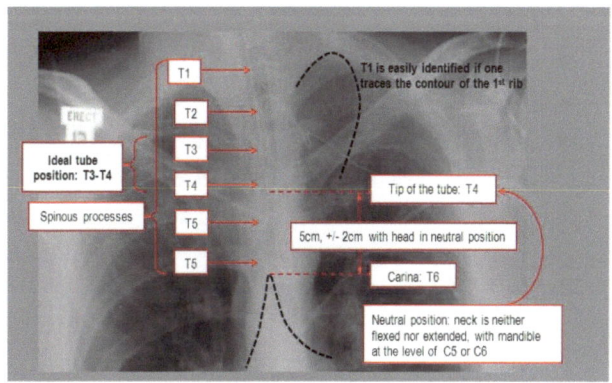

Image: www.derangedphysiology.com

End Tidal CO_2 (EtCO$_2$) Waveform Capnography
- Electronic device attached to the ETT to measure ETCO$_2$
- Displayed as a graph with a number value for ETCO$_2$ (see below)

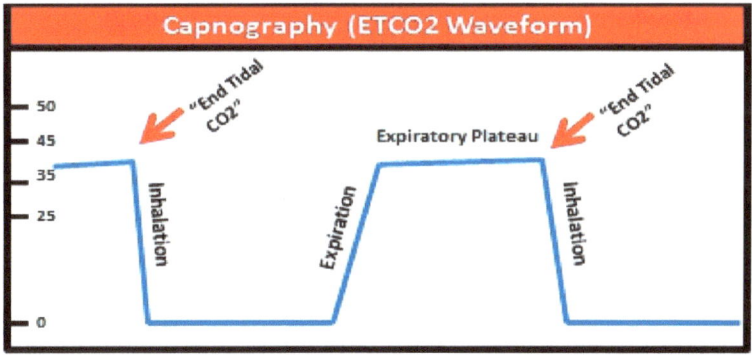

Colormetric Device
- Single use device that will change colors when CO_2 passes through it
    - Potential for false positives or malfunction of litmus paper
    - Provides no numerical value of the ETCO$_2$
- Device should be purple upon opening the package and should change to yellow if ET tube is correctly placed in the trachea
    - "Yellow is yes, purple is pull"

Rapid Sequence Intubation (RSI) & Pharmacology

- Involves co-administration of sedatives and neuromuscular blockades
- Indications and complications of intubation still apply
- Oxygenation and stabilization
- Proper medications should be used
    - Sedate to intubate is not the same as RSI
        - Increased risk of failure due to intact reflexes

7 P's for RSI Success
- **P**reparation
    - Make sure equipment is serviceable
        - Monitor pulse oximetry >93 %
        - Monitor blood pressure >100 mmHg
        - Cardiac monitor
        - $EtCO_2$ capnography
        - 1+ large bore IV line(s) [consider IO or cenral line]
        - BVM, suction, OG/NG tube
        - Laryngoscopy w/ back up device
        - Appropriately sized ETT w/ 10 mL syringe
        - All medications prepared
        - PATIENT POSITIONING
- **P**reoxygenate
    - 3-5 minutes, passive oxygenation via NC or NRM 10-15+ LPM
    - 8 vital capacity breaths with BVM at 15 LPM
- **P**retreatment
    - Stabilize vitals
- **P**aralysis with induction
    - Induction agent, paralytic, and pain control
- **P**rotect and position
    - Ear to sternal notch, ramping, pad behind shoulders for pediatrics
- **P**lacement with proof
    - Visual confirmation, capnography, chest x-ray
- **P**ost intubation management
    - Maintain sedation and pain control, oxygenation, etc.

Analgesics

Fentanyl (Duragesic, Actiq)
Opioid analgesic, 81x more powerful than morphine
- Dose based on intended use
    - 1 mcg/kg
    - Onset within 3-5 minutes, 30 – 60 minute duration
- Use with caution in patients with hypotension
    - Low risk of chest wall rigidity, but can be of concern
- Often requires an antiemetic
    - 4mg ondansetron (Zofran) or 25mg promethazine (Phenergan)
    - Naloxone (Narcan) 0.4-2 mg is the reversal agent

Induction Agents

Etomidate (Amidate)
Induction agent, preferred for awake sedation
- Fast onset, short half-life
    - 0.3 mg/kg
    - 15-45 second onset, 3-12 minute duration
- Use caution in hemodynamically unstable patients
- NO ANALGESIC PROPERTIES
- Can have vomiting when waking up
- Contraindications: Patients with adrenal suppression
    - Avoid in shock patients (especially septic shock) or Addison's disease
    - Avoid in COPD and asthmatic patients

Ketamine (Ketalar)
Hypnotic, analgesic, and amnestic properties
- Has the unique ability to preserve laryngeal reflexes (helps with airway protection)
- Dosage varies based on intended use
    - 1-2 mg/kg IV (RSI)
    - 0.1-0.2 mg/kg (Pain)
    - 5 mg/kg IM (Combative)
    - 40-60 second onset, 10-20 minute duration
    - Used to stop pain impulses
        - NMBs and Etomidate do not control pain
    - Potent bronchodilator (beta 2)
        - Preferred for RSI of asthmatic patients or those with reactive airway complications
    - Potential for increased secretions

- o Ketamine may cause laryngospasm
  - Suction *and if unresolved*
    - o 0.01 mg/kg IV Atropine *or*
    - o 0.4mg IV Scopolamine *slowly*
  - May hallucinate upon awakening
  - Can also be given intraosseous (IO) and Intranasal (IN)

Midazolam (Versed)
Benzodiazepine used for sedation/anxiolysis with anterograde amnesia
- "Helps you forget the event ever happened"
  - o Also used in seizures
- Dose varies based on intended use
  - o 2.5 to 5 mg IV
  - o 30-60 second onset, 15-30 minute duration
- Use lowest dose possible
- Do not combine with other benzodiazepine medications
- Flumazenil (Romazicon) 0.2mg is the reversal agent
  - o Note: flumazenil will adversely affect blood pressure

Propofol (Diprivan)
Hypnotic with no analgesic properties
- "Milk of Amnesia"
- Dose varies based on intended use
  - o 1-2 mg/kg IV
    - 25-50 mcg/kg/min (maintenance)
  - o 15-45 second onset, 5-10 minute duration
- Decreases cerebral perfusion pressure (CPP) and mean arterial pressure (MAP)
  - o Use with caution in the patients with a head injury
- Not a good choice for patients that are hemodynamically unstable
  - o Ketamine is a safer induction agent in shocky patients

Neuromuscular Blocking Agents (NMBAs)

Succinylcholine (Anectine)
Depolarizing Neuromuscular Blocking Agent
- Causes fasciculations (muscle twitching)
  - o Dose: 1-2 mg/kg
  - o < 1 minute onset, 4-6 minute duration
- Can cause hyperkalemia

- **Contraindications:** crush injuries, eye injuries, narrow-angle glaucoma, history of Malignant Hyperthermia (MH), burns > 24 hours old, hyperkalemia, or any nervous system disorder (ex. Guillain-Barre, Myasthenia gravis)
- **Malignant Hyperthermia (MH)**
    - Can be seen after the administration of succinylcholine (and gas anesthesia)
        - This is caused by a defect in the skeletal muscle sarcoplasmic reticulum
        - MH is due to a problem with calcium removal from the cell
    - Signs & Symptoms of MH:
        - Masseter spasm / trismus (lockjaw)
        - Sustained tetanic muscle contractions
        - Rapid increase in temperature (can become as high as 110°)
        - Increased $ETCO_2$
        - Tachycardia & hypertension
        - Mixed acidosis (hyperthermia)
    - Treat with Dantrolene Sodium (Dantrium)
        - Dose 2.5 mg/kg Rapid IV Bolus
        - DO NOT give calcium channel blockers (verapamil, diltiazem, amlodipine, etc.)

Rocuronium (Zemuron)
Non-Depolarizing Neuromuscular Blocking Agent
- Does not cause fasciculations
- < 2min onset (4-6 min), longer duration of action (30-60 min)
    - 0.6 -1.2 mg/kg
    - Maintenance: 0.1-0.2 mg/kg IV q20-30 min
- Sugammadex (Bridion) 16mg/kg used for immediate reversal of rocuronium

Vecuronium (Norcuron)
Non-Depolarizing Neuromuscular Blocking (NMB) agents
- Does not cause fasciculations
- Used post-succinylcholine or rocuronium to keep the patient paralyzed
    - Does not provide pain management
- Onset 90 – 120 seconds, longer duration of action (60-75 min)
    - 0.15 mg/kg
    - Maintenance: 0.01-0.1 mg/kg
- Does not require refrigeration
    - May be supplied as a powder that needs reconstitution

Protect the Airway
- Suction
- Secure
    - Per your program's protocols

Post-Intubation Management

Fentanyl: 0.5 – 1.5 mcg/kg IV – May repeat every 5 min
Ketamine: 0.5-1mg/kg IV – May repeat every 15min
Midazolam: 2 -5 mg IV - May repeat every 15 min

Post Intubation Management Infusions
- Fentanyl 1-3mcg/kg/hr
    - Mix 500mcg/ 100ml (5mcg/ml)
- Ketamine 1-2mg/kg/hr
    - Mix 500mg/250ml (2mg/ml)
- Midazolam .0.05-0.1mg/kg/hr
    - Mix 20mg/100ml (0.2mg/ml)

Richmond Agitation – Sedation Scale
- Mainly used in mechanically ventilated patients to avoid over or under-sedation
- Developed by critical care physicians, nurses, and pharmacists
- This is just one tool you can utilize to assess your patient's level of sedation

Score	Term	Description
+4	Combative	Overtly combative or violent and an immediate danger to staff
+3	Very agitated	Pulls on or removes tube(s) or catheter(s) or has aggressive behavior toward staff
+2	Agitated	Frequent nonpurposeful movement or patient ventilator dyssynchrony
+1	Restless	Anxious or apprehensive but movements not aggressive or vigorous
0	Alert and calm	
-1	Drowsy	Not fully alert but has sustained (> 10 seconds) awakenings, with eye contact, to voice
-2	Light sedation	Briefly (< 10 seconds) awakens with eye contact to voice
-3	Moderate sedation	Any movement (but no eye contact) to voice
-4	Deep sedation	No response to voice, but any movement to physical stimuli
-5	Unarousable	No response to voice or physical stimulation

Source: Crit Care © 2008 BioMed Central, Ltd.

RSI Checklist

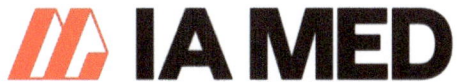

555 W 5TH ST, FLOOR 35
LOS ANGELES, CA 90013
(844) GO-IAMED   IAMED.US

IA MED RSI CHECKLIST	CHECK
PREOXYGENATE	
Oxygen tank >1000psi, Wall O_2 available	
HFNC, NRB, CPAP, BiPAP, BVM applied for oxygenation	
De-nitrogenation for 3min (Nitrogen Washout)	
Suction checked, working and on, backup available	
IV MEDICATIONS	
IV access available w/ fluids running	
NIBP, Consider hemodynamics	
PRE-TREATMENT ANALGESIA (dose, draw, confirm)	
INDUCTION AGENT (dose, draw, confirm)	
PARALYTIC AGENT (dose, draw, confirm)	
CONSIDER: Consider Fluids or Push Dose Pressor for hemodynamic compromise	
POST INTUBATION AGENTS (dose, draw, confirm)	
AIRWAY EQUIPMENT	
NPA or OPA available	
BVM (O_2, PEEP valve, Inline $ETCO_2$ attached)	
Direct Visual laryngoscopy equipment prepared: handle, blade size chosen, light operational	
Video Assisted Laryngoscopy equipment prepared: powers on, blade size chosen	
ETT Size chosen for patient (peds: age in years + 16 / 4)	
Stylet or Bougie available	
Tube Securing option available	
Supraglottic Airway Available (Combitube, King, LMA, iGel)	
Surgical Airway Available	
PATIENT	
Oxygenation >93%	
Positioning (ear to sternal notch/ramp)	
ECG/ NIBP/ SPO_2/ $ETCO_2$ visible on monitor	
TIME OUT	
Roles are assigned and understood	
PRE RSI-Medications Briefed	
Anticipated Problems Briefed	
POST RSI Care Briefed	

PRACTICAL, INSPIRING MEDICAL EDUCATION

Ventilator Patient Management

Lung Volumes Definitions

Tidal Volume (Vt)
- How much air the patient breathes in a normal breath
  - Excessive tidal volume can cause Ventilator-Induced Lung Injury (VILI)

Inspiratory Reserve Volume (IRV)
- The amount of air that can be forcefully inhaled in addition to a normal tidal volume breath

Expiratory Reserve Volume (ERV)
- The amount of air that can be forcefully exhaled after a normal tidal volume breath

Vital Capacity (VC)
- Tidal Volume + Inspiratory Reserve Volume + Expiratory Reserve Volume

Residual Volume (RV)
- The amount of air left in the respiratory tract following forceful exhalation

Total Lung Capacity (TLC)
- Inspiratory Reserve Volume + Tidal Volume + Expiratory Reserve Volume + Residual Volume

Dead Space
- The surfaces of the airway that are not involved in gaseous exchange
  - Gas exchange ONLY occurs in the alveoli
  - Dead Space Formula = **2ml/kg**

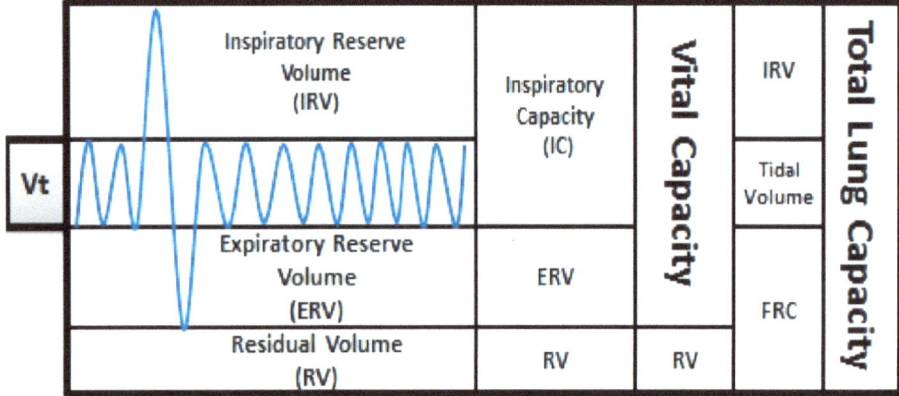

Chemoreceptors

Central
- Located in the medulla/pons
- Response is driven by **CO_2** and H⁺ levels in cerebral spinal fluid (CSF)
    - This is a slowly responding system

Peripheral
- Located in the aortic arch/carotid bodies
    - Response is driven by **O_2**, CO_2, H⁺

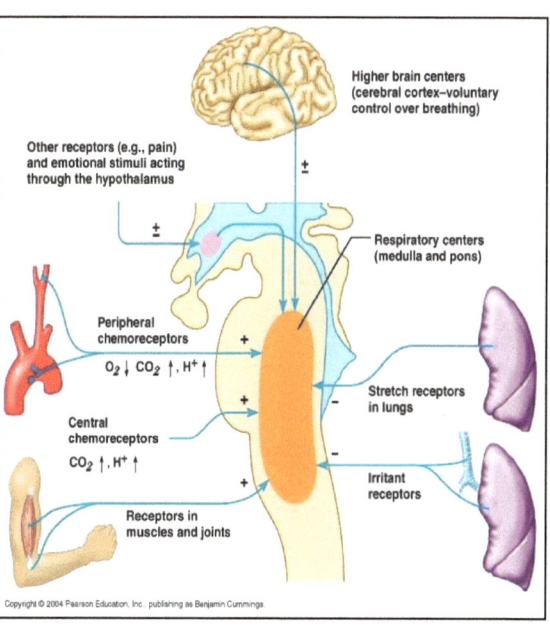

Ventilator Pearls
- Gold Standard for oxygenation – pulse oximetry (SpO₂)
- Gold Standard for ventilation – capnography (ETCO₂)

These two concepts will help you decide best approach for managing ventilator settings

Hypoxic Respiratory Failure
Inability to diffuse **O_2**

- ARDS, Pneumonia, CHF
- Evidenced by low pO₂ **< 60 mmHg**
- Treatment - ↑ **O_2 concentration (FiO₂) and PEEP**
    - Treatment assumes adequate tidal volume and rate have been maintained

> Tip: Increasing FiO₂, PEEP, or a combination of the two will increase oxygen saturations. Rate and tidal volume (Vt) will have minimal to no impact.

Hypercarbic Respiratory Failure
Inability to remove **CO_2**

- Damage to pons or upper medulla
    - Stroke & trauma
- Evidenced by respiratory acidosis
    - EtCO₂ > 45 mmHg
- Treatment- ↑ **tidal volume (Pplat), then ↑ rate**
    - Double Minute Volume (Ve), normal 4-8 L/min

NOTE: Use caution exceeding 8ml/kg of ideal body weight (IBW) for tidal volume settings (can cause VILI). If patient is receiving adequate tidal volumes (Plat 25 – 30 mmHg) begin to slowly increase the rate (F) to achieve a Ve of 4-8 L/min, and reassess every 15 minutes for improvement.

Ventilator Settings & Modes

Ventilator Settings

Tidal Volume (Vt)
4-8 cc/kg IBW (ideal body weight)

- Males: IBW = 50 kg + 2.3 kg for each inch over 5'
- Females: IBW = 45.5 kg + 2.3 kg for each inch over 5'
- The volume of air delivered per breath
- Excessive tidal volume can lead to Ventilator-Induced Lung Injury (VILI)

Rate (F)
12-20/min
- How many times a minute the patient is breathing (respiratory rate)

Minute Volume (Ve)
F x Vt (4-8 L/min)
- How much air is breathed by the patient in one minute

Inspiratory: Expiratory Ratio (I:E)
- The ratio of inspiration vs. expiration (1:2 = 1 second : 2seconds)
    - it takes longer to exhale

Fraction of Inspired Oxygen (FIO$_2$)
0.21 to 1.0
- Allows for very precise delivery of oxygen concentrations
    - 21% - 100% O$_2$ concentration
    - Measuring oxygen with liters per minute (lpm) is much less accurate

ALS & CRITICAL CARE

Positive End Expiratory Pressure (PEEP)
0-20 cm H_2O
- PEEP is what keeps the alveoli open so that oxygen can diffuse
- Adequate PEEP, increased FRC, and driving pressure helps prevent atelectasis (alveolar collapse), by reopening and stabilizing collapsed or unstable alveoli

Ventilator Delivery Methods

Volume (Tidal Volume)
- A preset tidal volume is delivered
- Once tidal volume is delivered the exhalation begins
- Volumes are consistent breath to breathe
- **Pressures are continuously monitored**

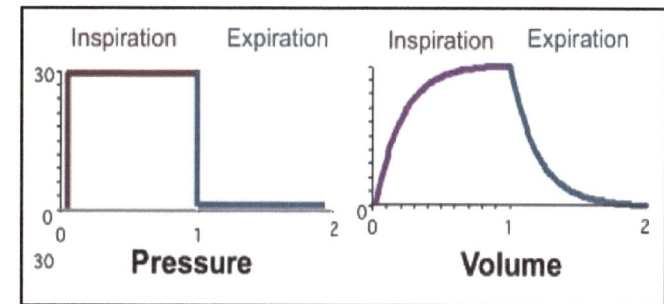

Pressure (Pressure Control)
- A preset inspiratory pressure is delivered
- Once pressure is achieved the exhalation begins
- Volumes are dynamic from breath to breath
- **Volumes need to be continuously monitored**

Resistance and Compliance

Peak Inspiratory Pressure (PIP)
<**35** cmH$_2$O
- Amount if resistance to overcome the ventilator circuit, any appliances, the ETT, and the main airways

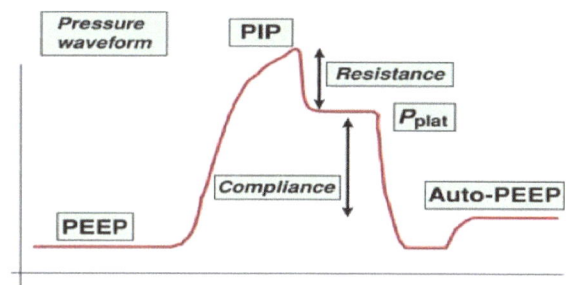

Plateau Pressure (Pplat)
<**30** cmH$_2$O
- This is a measurement of the pressure applied during positive pressure ventilations to the small airways and alveoli
  - Represents the static end inspiratory recoil pressure of the respiratory system, lung and chest wall respectively
- Measured during an inspiratory pause (i-hold) while on mechanical ventilation

Ventilator Modes

Controlled *Mandatory* Ventilation (CMV)
- Used in sedated, apneic or paralyzed patients
- Sometimes referred to as Continuous Mandatory Ventilation
- All breaths are triggered, limited, and cycled by the ventilator
    - Patient has NO ability to initiate their own breaths
    - If the patient tries to take a breath in this mode they later describe it "like sucking on an empty bottle."
        - Example: SAVe Ventilator

Assist-Control Ventilation (AC)
- The trigger for delivery of a breath can be either the patient or elapsed time
    - Preferred mode for patients with respiratory distress
- Ventilator supports every breath, whether it's initiated by the patient or the ventilator
    - Full tidal volume (Vt) *regardless* of respiratory effort or drive
- Used in Acute respiratory distress syndrome (ARDS), paralyzed or sedated patients
- Anxious patients who frequently trigger the ventilator can hyperventilate
    - Leads to "breath stacking" or "**auto-PEEP**"
        - Predisposes to barotrauma
        - Predisposes hemodynamic compromises
        - Diminishes the efficiency of the force generated by respiratory muscles
        - Increases the work of breathing
        - Increases the effort to trigger the ventilator
- Risk of Ventilator-Induced Lung Injury (VILI)

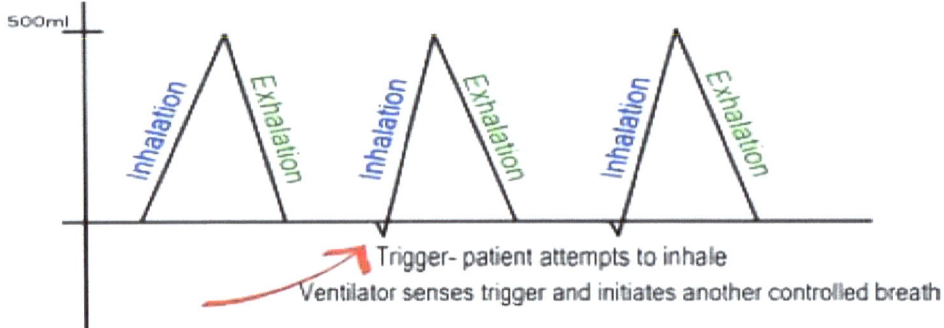

Synchronized Intermittent *Mandatory* Ventilation (SIMV)
- Assisted mechanical ventilation synchronized with the patient's breathing
    - The ventilator senses the patient taking a breath, then delivers a breath
- Spontaneous breathing by the patient occurs between the assisted mechanical breaths, which occur at preset intervals
    - If the patient fails to take a breath the ventilator will provide a mechanical breath
- Preferred for patients with an intact respiratory drive

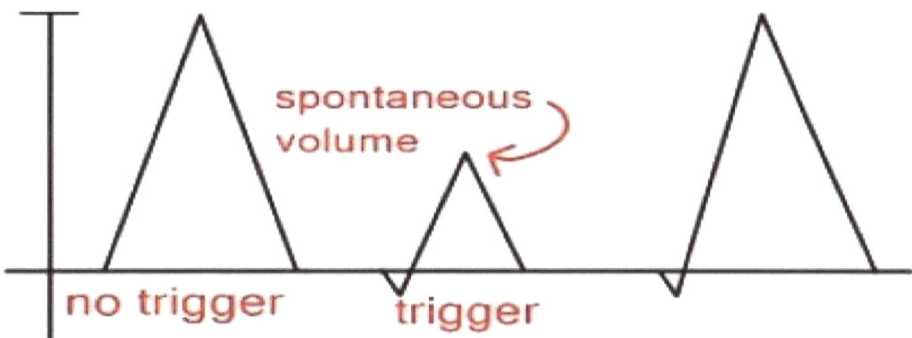

Pressure Support Ventilation (PSV)
- Pressure support makes it easier for the patient to overcome the resistance of the ET tube and is often used during weaning because it reduces the work of breathing
    - "Supports" or provides pressure during inspiration to decrease patient's overall work of breathing
- Patient determines tidal volumes, rate (minute volume)
- Requires consistent ventilatory effort by the patient

CPAP/BPAP

The ventilator method is often chosen in order to decrease work of breathing and lessen the need for intubation. This mode can be used on intubated patients as well.

Continuous Positive Airway Pressure (CPAP)
- The use of continuous positive pressure to maintain a continuous level of PEEP
- CPAP uses mild air pressure to keep an airway open

Bi-Level Continuous Positive Airway Pressure (BPAP)
- Uses alternating levels of PEEP to maintain oxygenation through pressure support during inhalation and exhalation, commonly used in pneumonia, COPD, asthma
- The term BiPAP™ refers to a specific manufacturer, not a vent setting

Ventilator Alarms

"DOPES" Ventilator Alarm Pneumonic
- **D**islodged — low pressure alarm
- **O**bstructed — high pressure alarm
- **P**neumothorax — high pressure alarm
- **E**quipment — machine failure, dead batteries, etc.
- **S**tacked breaths — high pressure alarm

Low Pressure
- Patient disconnection from machine (most common cause)
- Chest tube leaks
- Circuit leaks
- Airway leaks
- Hypovolemia

High Pressure
- Kinked line (most common cause)
- Coughing
- Secretions or mucus in the airway
- Patient biting the tube
- Reduced lung compliance (Pneumothorax, ARDS)
- Increased airway resistance

Patient - Ventilator Dyssynchrony
Respiratory demands not being met
- Inadequate pain control
- Inadequate sedation
- Curare Cleft

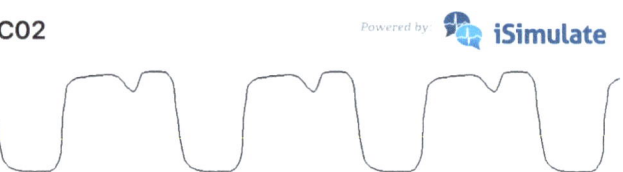

Effect on Patient
- Increased work of breathing
- Increased oxygen demand
- Increase heart rate
- Increase in BP
- Can lead to increase in ICP (especially concerning in TBI with increased ICP/CVAs)

Treatment:
- Manage Auto-PEEP
- Adjust sensitivity
- Adjust rate (match pt. demand)
- Adjust Minute Volume (Rate x VT)
- Suction
- Administer analgesia and sedation
    - Ketamine, fentanyl, midazolam

Troubleshooting the Ventilator

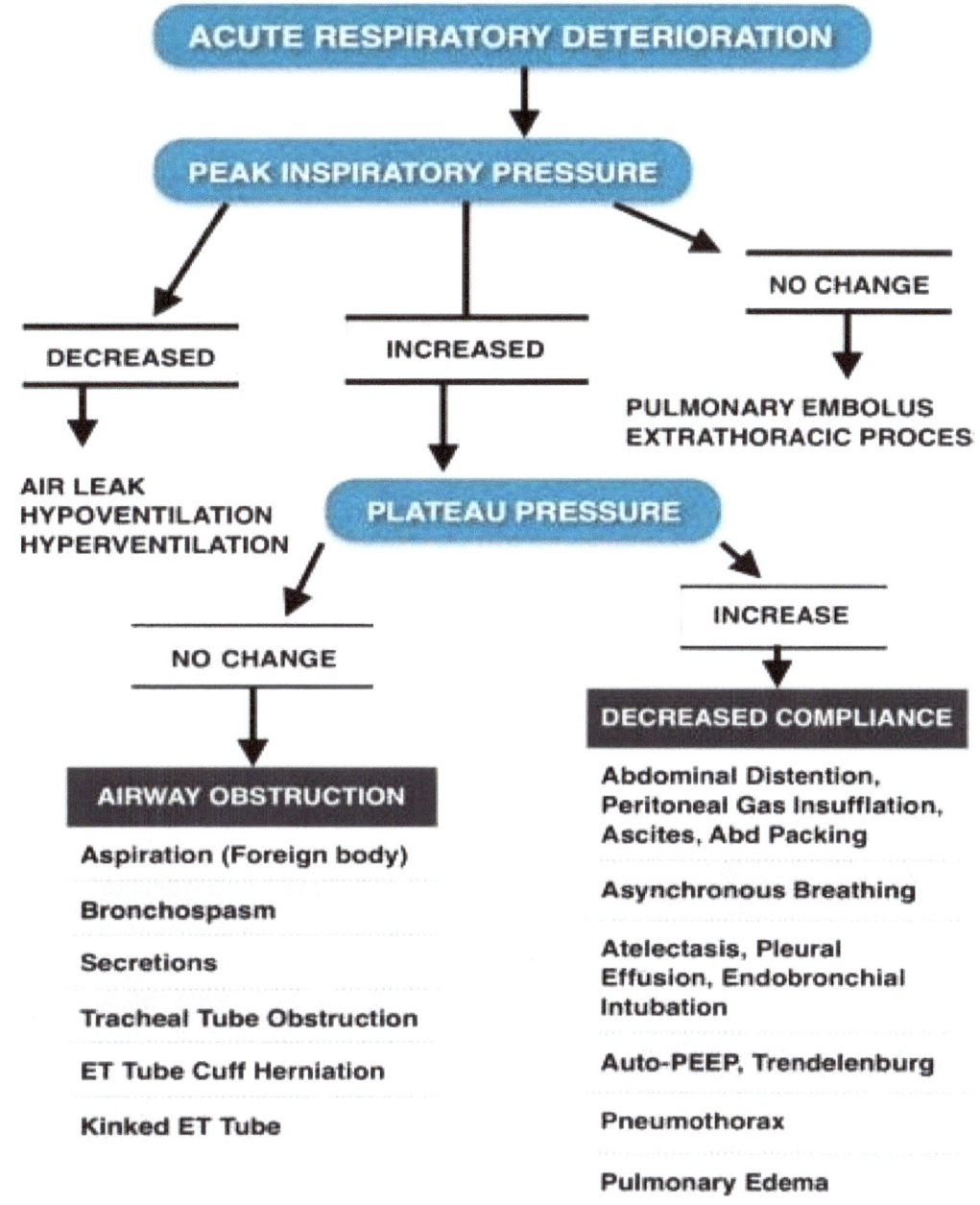

Cardiac Patients

Cardiac Responses
- In response to a decreased contractility, HR decreases
- In response to hypoxia, pulmonary arteries constrict (pulmonary hypertension)
- In response to a decrease in systemic perfusion, blood vessels constrict
    - Except in neurogenic (distributive), spinal, septic, and anaphylactic shock!
- A systemic decrease in vasoconstriction will decrease CO

Cardiac Output
CO (Cardiac Output) = HR x SV (Normal 4-8 L/min)
Normal Cardiac Index (2.5- 5 L/min)
    Assessment of the cardiac output based on the patient's size (BSA)

Dependent on:
- Preload
- Afterload
- Stroke Volume
- Contractility

Pulmonary Vascular Resistance
- Measures afterload of the Right Heart
- Normal (50-250 dynes)
- Increased PVR
    - Acidosis, Hypercapnia, Hypoxia, Atelectasis, ARDS
- Decreased PVR
    - Alkalosis, Hypocapnia, Vasodilating drugs

Systemic Vascular Resistance
- Measures afterload of the Left Heart
- Normally 800-1200 dynes
- Increased SVR:
    - Hypothermia, hypovolemic shock, decreased CO
- Decreased SVR:
    - Anaphylaxis, neurogenic shock, septic shock, vasodilating drugs

Cardiac Pharmacology

ACLS Drugs

Drug	Indication	Dosage
Adenosine	Narrow Complex SVT	6mg / 12mg
Amiodarone	V/F & Pulseless V tach	300mg 1st dose / 150mg 2nd dose
Atropine	Sinus Bradycardia & Organophosphate Poisoning	0.5mg q3min (max 3mg)
Dopamine	2nd Line for Bradycardia & Hypotension (<70 SBP)	2-20mcg / kg / min
Defibrillation	V/F & Pulseless V tach	120J then 200J Biphasic or 200J then 360J Monophasic
Epinephrine	VF / Pulseless VT / Asystole / PEA	1mg (1:10,000) q3-5min
Lidocaine	Alternative to Amiodarone	1.0 - 1.5 mg / kg (max 3mg / kg)
Magnesium Sulfate	Torsades De Pointe & Arrhythmia 2° to Digitalis	1 - 2 grams (over 30 - 60 min)

Neurovascular System Refresher
- α_1 - Vasoconstrict
- β_1 - Increase heart rate & contractility
- β_2 - Dilate bronchioles & blood vessels
- Dopaminergic – Gut kidney vessel dilation
- Cholinergic – Decrease heart rate

Mnemonic: You have one heart and two lungs: β_1 affects the heart, β_2 affects the lungs

Inotropic and Vasopressor agents
- Phenylephrine (Neo-Synephrine)
  - α-agonist
- Norepinephrine/Epinephrine
  - both α-agonist and some β-agonist activity
  - Potent vasoconstriction and positive inotropic effects
- Dopamine
  - Dose dependent
  - Higher doses it acts as an α-agonist causing vasoconstriction

- Dobutamine
    - Positive inotropic agent – improves contractility
    - Used in patients with low CI and high PAWP with SBP above 80
- Milrinone
    - Positive inotropic effect and vasodilation

TIP:
Norepinephrine and dopamine are often used in **hypovolemic shock**
Both dobutamine and milrinone are often used in **cardiogenic shock**

SVR and Preload Pharmacology

Medications that affect Systemic Vascular Resistance (SVR)
- Increase SVR
    - Dopamine, phenylephrine (Neo-Synephrine), epinephrine, norepinephrine (Levophed)
    - Norepinephrine - used for patients in profound hypotension
- Decrease SVR
    - Nitroprusside (Nipride), High Dose NTG, CCBs, ACEi, α Blockers, Dobutrex, Natrecor
    - Nitroprusside (Nipride) - reduces preload and afterload by dilation (can cause cyanide toxicity)
        - *This is not the same as nitroglycerine*
    - Nicardipine – reduces afterload (does not cause cyanide toxicity)

Medications that Affect Cardiac Preload
- Increase preload
    - Vasoconstrictors (drugs that also increase SVR), fluids
- Decrease preload
    - Vasodilators, Morphine, Lasix, Nitro (drugs that decrease SVR)

↑ SVR *Vasoconstrictors*	↓ SVR *Vasodilators*	↑ Preload *Vasoconstrictors*	↓ Preload *Vasodilators*
Dopamine Phenylephrine Epinephrine Norepinephrine	Nitroprusside Nicardipine High Dose Nitro CCBs	Dopamine Phenylephrine Epinephrine Norepinephrine Fluids	Morphine Lasix Nitroglycerine

Shock Management
- Volume
  - Affects preload and contractility
- Ventilation
  - Maximize oxygen delivery
- Vasopressors
  - Consider epinephrine or norepinephrine for non-cardiac related causes of shock
  - Consider Dopamine or Dobutamine for cardiac related causes of shock

Conclusion

Prior planning and use of forward thinking will make the commercial transfer of your advanced or critical care patient seamless. Being familiar and comfortable with your equipment takes a variable out of the equation to ease your patient care.

While it is imperative that you are always re-assessing your patient's airway during transport, it is best to manage it prior to leaving the discharge facility. Use the resources available prior to leaving the hospital team.

Always refer to your protocols for medications carried, indications and dosages. The examples in this chapter may not pertain to your program

While some of the information discussed may be new to you, always refer to your program's scope of practice and conduct independent research as a medical professional to ensure you continue to provide safe, competent care to your patients.

QUICK REFERENCE CHARTS

Ventilator Setting	Normal Value
Vt (Tidal Volume)	4-8ml/kg
F (Rate)	12-20/min
Ve (Minute Volume)	F x Vt (4-8 L/min)
I:E (Inspiratory: Expiratory ratio)	1:2
FiO2 (Fraction of Inspired Oxygen)	0.21 to 1.0 (21% - 100%)
Pplat (Plateau Pressure)	<30 cmH$_2$O
PEEP (Positive End Expiratory	0-20 cmH$_2$O
PFR (Peak Flow Rate)	60 LPM

Oxygen Adjustment Calculation	(FiO$_2$ x P1) / P2
Torr Values	
Sea Level	760 torr (1 ATM)
18k MSL	380 torr (1/2 ATM)

AMI Locations "PAILS"	EKG Leads	Vessel	Treatment
Posterior	Reciprocal changes in V1,V2,V3,V4	LCX	MONA
Anterior	V2, V3, V4	LAD	MONA
Inferior	II, III, aVF	RCA	Fluids (no nitro/Beta Blockers)
Lateral	1, V5, V6, aVL	LCX	MONA
Septal	V1, V2	LAD	MONA

Note: Posterior and Lateral MIs can be caused by either LCX or RCA occlusion

Anion Gap Acidosis Cause	Offending Agent	Treatment
Methanol	Methyl Alcohol, Wood Alcohol, Sterno	IV Ethanol or Fomepizole
Uremia	Kidney failure	Dialysis
DKA	Diabetic Ketoacidosis	IV Fluid Resuscitation/Insulin
Propylene Glycol	Liquid agent used in Diazepam/Lorazepam	Flumazenil (Romazicon)
Isoniazid (INH) **I**ron	Tuberculosis medication Iron supplements	Pyridoxine (Vitamin B6) Deferoxamine
Lactate	From anaerobic metabolism	Correct inadequate tissue perfusion
Ethylene Glycol	Antifreeze	IV Ethanol or
Salicylates	Aspirin	Dialysis

Medical Emergency	Treatment
Diabetic Ketoacidosis (DKA)	IV Fluids/insulin
Hyperosmolar Non-Ketosis Hyperglycemia (HHNK)	IV Fluids/insulin
Syndrome of Inappropriate Anti-Diuretic Hormone (SIADH)	Hypertonic Saline
Diabetes Insipidus (DI)	Vasopressin/Desmopressin/DDAVP
Esophageal Varices	Somatostatin/Sandostatin/Octreotide
Mallory Weiss/Boerhaave's Tear	Supportive Care/EGD
Thyrotoxicosis/Graves's Disease	IV Fluids/ Beta Blocker/Dexamethasone/Tylenol
Hypothyroidism/Myxedema Coma	Levothyroxine (Synthroid)
Addison's Disease (Adrenal	Steroids
Liver Failure	Lactulose
Septic Shock	Treat underlying cause/ Levophed
Pancreatitis	Treat underlying cause/ Demerol for pain
Hyperkalemia	Albuterol, Bicarb, Insulin, Dextrose, Lasix, Kayexalate, Calcium Gluconate
Hypokalemia	Potassium

IA MED
LAB VALUE QUICK REFERENCE

Basic Metabolic Panel (BMP)

Sodium	135 – 145 mEq/L
Potassium	3.5 – 5.0 mEq/L
Chloride	96 – 106 mEq/L
Bicarbonate/Total CO_2	22 – 26 mEq/L
BUN	8 – 23 mEq/L
Creatinine	0.7 – 1.4 mg/dL
Glucose	70 – 110 mg/dL

Complete Blood Count (CBC)

RBC*	5 million/µL
Hemoglobin*	~15 g/dL
Hematocrit*	~45%
Platelet	150K – 400K/µL
WBC	4,500 – 11,000/µL

*Varies based on gender

Cardiac Enzyme Panel

Troponin I	< 0.04 ng/mL
Troponin T	< 0.01 ng/mL
CK	20 – 200 U/L
CK-MB	0 – 3 ng/mL
Myoglobin	5 – 70 ng/mL

Arterial Blood Gas

pH	7.35 – 7.45
PCO_2	35 – 45 mmHg
HCO_3	22 – 26 mmol/L
PO_2	80 – 100 mmHg
SaO_2	94 – 99%
BE	-2 – 2 mEq/L

Comprehensive Metabolic Panel (CMP)

Sodium	135 – 145 mEq/L
Potassium	3.5 – 5.0 mEq/L
Chloride	96 – 106 mEq/L
Bicarbonate/Total CO_2	22 – 26 mEq/L
BUN	8 – 23 mEq/L
Creatinine	0.7 – 1.4 mg/dL
Glucose	70 – 110 mg/dL
Calcium	8.5 – 10.2 mg/dL
Ionized Calcium	4.4 – 5.4 mg/dL
Albumin	3.5 – 5.5 g/dL
Total Protein	6.0 – 8.0 g/dL
ALP	45 – 115 U/L
ALT	7 – 55 U/L
AST	8 – 48 U/L
Bilirubin	0.1 – 1.2 mg/dL

Gastrointestinal Function Panel

Albumin	3.5 – 5.5 g/dL
Total Protein	6.0 – 8.0 g/dL
ALP	45 – 115 U/L
ALT	7 – 55 U/L
AST	8 – 48 U/L
Bilirubin	0.1 – 1.2 mg/dL
Amylase	25 – 125 U/L
Lipase	5 – 60 U/L

Coagulation Panel

PT	10 – 13 sec
PTT	25 – 40 sec
INR	0.9 – 1.3

PRACTICAL, INSPIRING MEDICAL EDUCATION

© 2020 Immediate Action Medicine, LLC

Pediatric Age Ranges	
Neonate	Birth to 28 days
Infant	29 days to one year
Toddler	One year to two years
Child	>Two Years old
Emergency Intervention Formulas	
ETT Diameter	(16 + Age)/4
	"2/3/4"
Suction/NG/Foley	**2** x ETT (i.e. 5mm ETT - 10fr Foley)
ETT insertion depth	**3** x ETT size (i.e. 5mm ETT - 15mm insertion depth)
Chest Tube	**4** x ETT (i.e. 5mm ETT - 20fr chest tube)
Normal BP	90 + (2 x Age)
Hypotensive BP	70 + (2 x Age)

Fluid Resuscitation (EMERGENCY)

Max of 2 bolus infusions

Neonate/Infant	10cc/kg
Toddler/Child	20cc/kg

Non-Emergent Fluid Maintenance
"4/2/1"

1-10 kg	**4**cc/kg/h
10-20 kg	**2**cc/kg/hr
>20 kg	**1**cc/kg/hr

Glucose Management

D-Stick <60mg/dL, All ages 2cc/kg

Neonate	D10
Infant	D25
Toddler/Child	D50

Toxic Agent	Antidote
Aspirin (ASA)	Bicarb
Benzodiazepines	Flumazenil (Romazicon)
Beta Blockers	Glucagon
Calcium Channel Blockers	Calcium Gluconate
Cocaine	Benzodiazepines
Crotalinae Snakes (Pit Vipers)	CroFab, FabAV
Cyanide	Amyl Nitrite, Sodium Nitrite, Sodium Thiosulfate
Digitalis	Digibind, Digoxin Fab
Phenytoin (Dilantin)	Supportive Care
Ethylene Glycol	IV Ethanol OR Fomepizole (Antizol)
Hydrocarbons	Intubate
Isoniazid (INH)	Pyridoxine (Vitamin B6)
Iron	Deferoxamine
Methanol	IV Ethanol OR Fomepizole (Antizol)
Opioids	Naloxone (Narcan)
Organophosphates	Atropine/2-Pam Chloride/ Benzos
Tricyclic Antidepressants	Bicarb
Acetaminophen (Tylenol)	Mucomyst/Acetadote

Fahrenheit	Celsius
105°	40.6°
104°	40.0°
103°	39.4°
102°	38.9°
101°	38.3°
100°	37.8°
99°	37.2°
98°	36.7°
97°	36.1°
96°	35.6°

MERCI TRAVEL CHECKLIST

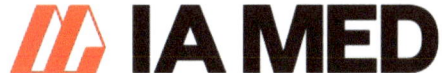

555 W 5TH ST, FLOOR 35
LOS ANGELES, CA 90013
(844) GO-IAMED   IAMED.US

Medical Escort & Repatriation Course, International: Travel Checklist

	Pre-Transport	Patient Transport	Post-Transport
Obtain updated medical report			
Airline, hotel, ground transport accommodations			
Medical kit/bag with mission specific items, including charger and POC batteries			
Support letter for TSA and other security/airline screenings			
Mobile phone with international access			
International power converter & charger; power bank			
Travel documents (passport, I.D., visas, vaccinations) with copies on mobile phone; professional licenses & certifications			
Aware of local customs/traditions			
Aware of drug/medication restrictions of countries visited			
Minimal jewelry and expensive clothes/luggage			
Travel insurance/personal liability insurance policy			
Weather appropriate clothing			
Bags packed per local airport requirements			
Confirm patient and travel companion travel documents in hand			
Assist/confirm patient and travel companion bags packed per airport requirements			
Retrieve any patient or travel companion checked bags at final destination			
Provide receiving facility or caretaker with a verbal and written report, including transport documentation/signatures			

FAA Packsafe: https://www.faa.gov/hazmat/packsafe/

WHO: https://www.who.int

CDC: https://wwwnc.cdc.gov/travel/notices

Embassies: http://www.embassyworld.com

PRACTICAL, INSPIRING MEDICAL EDUCATION

REVIEW QUESTIONS

1. While conducting a medical escort, it is not important to protect your patient's private information due to _____.
    a. International travel
    b. Commercial travel
    c. Low acuity of the patient
    d. Patient private information must always be protected

2. Which of the following is not routinely a part of a quality management system?
    a. Team member satisfaction
    b. Governmental compliance
    c. Patient care
    d. Customer satisfaction

3. There are several avenues medical escort/repatriation transfers come about. These include all of the following except:
    a. Private individuals
    b. Travel insurance or assistance companies
    c. Other air medical providers
    d. Hospitals and case managers
    e. 911 service

4. Customer service is a vital aspect of conducting commercial transfers because _____. [choose all that apply]
    a. The patient will remember your name
    b. The patient will report your services to their insurance company
    c. Your company will receive feedback on your services
    d. You will never see the patient again, it does not matter

5. Which of the following types of patients are not eligible for commercial transport?
    a. Ambulatory
    b. Cardiovascular collapse
    c. Surgically repaired hip fractures
    d. ECMO and external cardiac assistive devices

6. Of the following, who cannot decline your patient from being transported on the aircraft?
    a. The airline
    b. The captain
    c. You
    d. The wheelchair porter

7. Your program will define communication requirements while on a transfer. This can include: [select all that apply]
    a. Cellular phones with international coverage
    b. E-mail
    c. Texting/chat apps
    d. Safety updates

8. When traveling outside of your country of residence, it is important to _____.
    a. Understand local customs
    b. Visit as much of the city as possible
    c. Wear a lot of jewelry and expensive clothing
    d. Be adventurous with food

9. When traveling, always carry originals and digital copies of all of the following except:
    a. Relevant licenses/certifications
    b. Passport/Identification
    c. Immunizations
    d. Birth Certificate

10. Airline safety topics that you have control over include: [select all that apply]
    a. Luggage and allowed items
    b. Use of seat belts
    c. Safety around the aircraft
    d. Following rules and regulations of your home country
    e. Following all cabin crew directions

11. Under what circumstances could you be on an active airplane ramp or tarmac? [select all that apply]
    a. Emergency landing
    b. Tarmac transfer of your patient
    c. Boarding or deplaning
    d. Transport to and from the aircraft

12. If your aircraft makes an emergency landing, when should you notify your chain of command?
    a. As soon as reasonably practical
    b. After assessing all passengers for injury
    c. After unloading all luggage and belongings
    d. After assisting all other passengers evacuate

13. Which of the following is not a part of 'Just culture?'
    a. Safety reporting
    b. Preoccupation with failure
    c. Reluctance to simplify
    d. Sensitivity to operations
    e. Deference to expertise
    f. Resilience

14. Crew resource management, as it pertains to medical escorts and repatriations, is most heavily focused on Human Factors. Which of the following is NOT considered a part of Human Factors?
    a. Problem solving
    b. Decision making
    c. Weights and balances
    d. Communication

15. Situational awareness and forward thinking are pertinent during the commercial transfer of patients because _____: [Select all that apply]
    a. Of the low acuity of your patient
    b. They allow you to anticipate future needs
    c. They allow you to set up your work environment
    d. The cabin crew will ensure safety

16. Your ability to safely provide medical care and monitoring during commercial transfers can be impacted by which of the following: [select all that apply]
    a. Illness
    b. Medications
    c. Stress
    d. Fatigue

17. Stress and circadian rhythm imbalances contribute to fatigue by _____. [select all that apply]
    a. Disrupting your sleep/wake cycles
    b. Leading to poor dietary and lifestyle choices
    c. Prolonging physical or mental activity
    d. Causing irritability and depression

18. What is the first step in fatigue mitigation?
    a. Healthy sleep environment
    b. Eating nutritious foods
    c. Recognizing fatigue
    d. Keep a regular schedule

19. You are a single provider in the middle of a patient transfer from Los Angeles, CA to Mumbai, India. Before accepting the transfer, you worked three straight night shifts at your regular job. You now realize that you are fatigued. How do you best manage yourself?
    a. Go to sleep immediately so you can better function in a few hours
    b. Tell the cabin crew to monitor your patient so you can lay down a few rows back
    c. Eat and drink whatever you can to stay awake and monitor your patient
    d. Inform your patient, travel companion and cabin crew that you *may* close your eyes and to notify you of any patient needs

20. Which of the following does not lead to sleep deprivation?
    a. Rapid travel across multiple time zones
    b. Ensuring adequate rest
    c. Shift work
    d. Delayed sleep phase disorder

21. There are many causes of stress, both personal and professional. Which of the following is not a sign or symptom of stress?
    a. Increased motivation
    b. Headache
    c. Moodiness
    d. Elevated blood pressure

22. Which of the following is an example of how not to manage stress:
    a. Work on time management
    b. Learn how to say "no"
    c. Get adequate sleep
    d. Eat food that makes you happy

23. Using appropriate body mechanics is important not only for your safety, but your patient's safety. Which situation(s) requires the use of proper body mechanics when providing direct care? [select all that apply]
    a. Prolonged sitting
    b. Observing counter agents check-in bags
    c. Assisting your patient with transfers
    d. Assisting your patient with the administration of their medication

24. When transferring a patient from the bed to a wheelchair, which of the following is not a step:
    a. Use small steps when navigating to the wheelchair
    b. Place a sheet under the patient
    c. Bend the patient's knees
    d. Lift the patient straight up from the supine position

25. When transferring a patient from a wheelchair to a car, which of the following is not considered part of proper transfer procedure:
    a. Place your legs in between the patient's legs
    b. Lock the brakes
    c. Remove footrests
    d. Lower the patient into the vehicle while protecting their head

26. All blood and bodily fluids are considered _____.
    a. Infectious
    b. Dirty
    c. Without pathogens
    d. Safe

27. What two bloodborne pathogens are specifically discussed by OSHA? [select all that apply]
    a. Hepatitis C
    b. HIV/AIDS
    c. Hepatitis B
    d. Viral Meningitis
    e. A and D
    f. B and C

28. Which is an appropriate receptacle for sharps?
    a. The regular trash
    b. A red biohazard bag
    c. On the floor
    d. An impermeable container with a biohazard symbol

29. Which is the best, most reasonable method of preventing the transmission of bloodborne pathogens?
    a. Not coming in contact with bloodborne pathogens
    b. Handwashing
    c. Wearing appropriate PPE
    d. Wearing a mask

30. What is your first step if you have been exposed to a bloodborne pathogen or infectious disease?
    a. Complete an exposure report
    b. Seek medical attention
    c. Flush your eyes
    d. Remain calm and assess the situation

31. What is the purpose of Critical Incident Stress Debriefing or Management?
    a. To help deal with major or traumatic events
    b. Provide a review of your commercial transfer
    c. An intervention when fatigue sets in
    d. It allows you to share feedback on how the transfer could have been better

32. Which of the following is true regarding air circulation on board the commercial aircraft? [select all that apply]
    a. It moves from the rear to forward
    b. It is moves from the floor to the ceiling
    c. It is exchanged approximately 25 times per hour
    d. It is exchanged approximately 12 times per hour
    e. It is filtered through the HEPA filter approximately 12 times per hour
    f. It is filtered through the HEPA filter approximately 25 times per hour

33. Ride-share vehicles and taxis may _____.
    a. Have specific use policies by your program
    b. Be used interchangeably
    c. Never be used
    d. Be used exclusively

34. While transporting in a ground ambulance, safety for you and your patient are paramount. Which of the following is not allowed?
    a. Safety restraints for people and bags/equipment
    b. Medical escort operating the stretcher
    c. Lights and sirens use for threat to life or limb
    d. Use of seatbelts while caring for a patient

35. What considerations should not be made in the selection of ground transportation for your patient?
    a. Is the vehicle too low to the ground, making it difficult for them to get out?
    b. Is the vehicle too tall, making it difficult for them to get in?
    c. Is the vehicle large enough to accommodate all passengers and luggage?
    d. Fuel economy

36. Who has the ultimate responsibility to determine what medications and/or medical supplies are permitted into a country?
    a. The supervisor for the transport company
    b. The medical attendant in charge of the patient
    c. The Flight Coordinator
    d. The airline cabin crew

37. Which of the following is not a category of wheelchair assistance?
    a. WCHR
    b. WCHB
    c. WCHS
    d. WCHC

38. Your patient is receiving 4 LPM of oxygen on the ground (sea level) with saturations of 95% after the use of an incentive spirometer and cough/deep breathing. The patient's skin is color appropriate and denies difficulty breathing. Forward thinking and situational awareness show: [select all that apply]
    a. Likely unable to administer a high enough FiO2
    b. Dalton's law says the patient will require >4 LPM
    c. The patient is at risk of deterioration at altitude
    d. There are no issues with commercial transport of this patient.

39. You are transporting a 66 year old female who is currently 5 days postoperative from an uncomplicated (L) hip repair. Your patient is at high risk for:
    a. Myocardial infarction
    b. Deep vein thrombosis
    c. Foot drop
    d. Osteomyelitis

40. You are transporting a 66 year old female who is currently 5 days postoperative from an uncomplicated (L) hip repair, which medication is your patient most likely to be taking?
    a. Antipyretic medication
    b. Antihypertensive medication
    c. Anticoagulant medication
    d. Ace-inhibitor medication

41. What types of patients will require additional assistance to prevent skin breakdown?
    a. Limited mobility only
    b. Recent wrist surgery only
    c. Decreased sensorium only
    d. Using oxygen only
    e. (A) and (B)
    f. (C) and (D)
    g. (A) and (C)

42. While your patient's comfort is very important, their positioning (according to their clinical picture) is more important. Which of the following are appropriate positions for your CHF patient receiving 3 LPM of oxygen? [select all that apply]
    a. Upright
    b. Fully flat
    c. High fowlers
    d. Semi-fowlers

43. Which class of service will afford you more space that is conducive to a proper working environment?
    a. Business/First
    b. Economy
    c. Economy stretcher
    d. Private cabin

44. While loading your stretcher patient on the plane, you are not expected to _____.
    a. Direct the transfer process
    b. Monitor your patient's response to the transfer(s)
    c. Ensure your patient is secured on the aircraft
    d. Serve as a second set of eyes to the crew conducting the transfer

45. Upon checking in, you realize that you and the patient are not seated together. Which of the following is/are an appropriate next step. [select all that apply]
    a. Speak to counter agent
    b. Speak to gate agent
    c. Speak to lead cabin attendant
    d. Provide feedback to your flight coordinator

46. Which gas law is most responsible in explaining why supplemental oxygen may be required while transporting at altitude?
    a. Boyle's
    b. Charles
    c. Dalton's
    d. Fick's
    e. Henry's

47. You are transporting your patient at an altitude of 35,000'. You understand that the FiO2 of the ambient air is:
    a. 21%
    b. 25%
    c. 11%
    d. 18%

48. Which of the following is considered the physiologically deficient zone? FMP-FPHYS-1003
    a. 50k MSL - 80k MSL
    b. Sea level - 10k MSL
    c. 5k MSL - 10k MSL
    d. 10k MSL - 50k MSL

49. You are conducting a commercial transport. While at a cruising altitude of 30k ft. MSL your pilot announces that he is unable to maintain the cabin pressure and suspects a pressure leak. What is your expected TUC (Time of Useful Consciousness)? FMP-FPHYS-1005
    a. 90 sec
    b. 180 sec
    c. 45 sec
    d. 5 mins
    e. 10 mins

50. Which of the following **is not** affected by Boyle's Law
    a. Foley Catheter
    b. Pressure Bag
    c. ETT Cuff
    d. Bag of Saline
    e. Bowel obstruction

51. Which of the following occurs only in ascent? FMP-FPHYS-1016
    a. Barodontalgia
    b. Barosinusitis
    c. Barotitis Media
    d. Referred pain

52. Which of the following is not a type of Hypoxia?
    a. Stagnant
    b. Histotoxic
    c. Hypoxic
    d. Anemic
    e. Hypemic

53. Which of the following is a self-imposed stressor of flight?
    a. Dehydration
    b. Fatigue
    c. Noise
    d. Vibration

54. Generally speaking, as a flight crew member, how long after diving should you avoid flying? FMP-FPHYS-1023
    a. Zero
    b. 12 hours
    c. 36 hours
    d. 48 hours
    e. 24-48 hours

55. Which type of hypoxia is common during commercial flights, especially in the economy cabin?
    a. Hypoxic
    b. Stagnant
    c. Hypemic
    d. Histotoxic

56. You are transporting a patient on a pulse-dose portable oxygen concentrator (POC). You are monitoring their pulse oximetry as it correlates to their respiratory rate. Their pulse ox is below 90% and their intentional respiratory rate is approximately 24 per minute. What is your next best step?
    a. Coach them with their breathing and the POC
    b. Increase the setting
    c. Abort the transport
    d. Not to worry, it will be okay

57. Your patient will see the greatest amount of changes from _____.
    a. 1k - 5k ft MSL
    b. 6k - 10k ft MSL
    c. 10k - 20k ft MSL
    d. 20k - 25k ft MSL

58. In the event that your patient has a medical emergency on board, it is important to: [select all that apply]
    a. Stay calm
    b. Care for your patient within your protocols & resources available
    c. Notify the cabin crew
    d. Discuss with MedLink/MedAire/STAT-MD
    e. Use effective communication

59. In the event of a medical emergency mid-flight, which of the following agencies on the ground might you or the crew speak with regarding the patient's condition?
    a. AirLink/AireMed
    b. MedAire/MedLink/STAT-MD
    c. MedAdvice/GroundMed
    d. AirLink/LinkMed

60. Which of the following portions of the obstetric history should you obtain for pregnant patients? [select all that apply]
    a. Gravida
    b. Term births
    c. Preterm births
    d. Abortions
    e. Living children

61. What are some of the normal assessment findings of the neonate? [select all that apply]
    a. Cricoid ring is the narrowest part of airway
    b. Manage thermoregulation well
    c. Heart rate 120-160
    d. Low oxygen demand

62. When rapidly assessing the pediatric patient, which mnemonic applies?
    a. TICLS
    b. PICLS
    c. NICLS
    d. SICLS

63. The pediatric airway is more fragile due to: [select all that apply]
    a. Smaller lower airways
    b. Lower aspiration risk
    c. Highly reactive airways
    d. Higher compensatory methods

64. What would the rate of maintenance fluid be for a 25 kg child? FMP-PEDEM-1014
    a. 65 ml/hr
    b. 85 ml/hr
    c. 75 ml/hr
    d. 125 ml/hr

65. Which of the following is a sign that is **not** associated with Cushing's Triad?
    a. Irregular Respirations
    b. Bradycardia
    c. Hypertension
    d. Hypotension

66. Which of the following findings are associated with increasing ICP? [select all that apply]
    a. Decreased level of consciousness
    b. Pupillary changes
    c. Posturing
    d. Changes in vital signs

67. You arrive at the discharge facility to transport a patient who is positive for a Kernig's sign and Brudzinki's sign. Which of the following conditions do you suspect the patient is suffering from? FMP-NEURO-1022
    a. Meningitis
    b. Encephalopathy
    c. Encephalitis
    d. Splenic laceration

68. Your patient was involved in a motor vehicle collision 10 days prior to transfer. They have an incomplete spinal injury. You expect them to present with:
    a. No sensation below the injury
    b. No proprioception below the injury
    c. Some sensation below the injury
    d. No motor below the injury

69. You are transporting a 42 y/o male with a diagnosis of schizophrenia. You are halfway through a 12 hour flight when you notice he begins to get agitated. Your first intervention is:
    a. Therapeutic communication
    b. Non-pharmacological restraints
    c. Pharmacologic restraints
    d. Notify the cabin crew

70. Which of the following medications is not appropriate in the management of an acutely psychotic patient?
    a. Ketorolac
    b. Diphenhydramine
    c. Haloperidol
    d. Lorazepam

71. When treating a patient suspected of having a pulmonary embolism you suspect the patient's hypoxemia is caused by which of the following mechanisms?
    a. V/Q (Ventilation/Perfusion) Mismatch
    b. Loss of cardiac preload
    c. Increase in pulmonary vascular resistance
    d. Cardiogenic shock

72. You are transporting an 85 y/o female with a diagnosis of pneumonia. She is on appropriate oral antibiotics, steroids, and bronchodilators. She is receiving setting 4 on the portable oxygen concentrator with a pulse ox of 95%. She complains of sudden onset shortness of breath with the following vitals: 102/55, 120 HR, 28 RR, 86% SpO2, 38 temp. While reaching for her MDI, she slumps in her seat. When performing basic airway management, what is important to remember?
    a. Airway adjuncts are not important
    b. An adequate mask seal is not important
    c. Only enough of a bag squeeze for adequate chest rise
    d. 24 breaths per minute

73. Your patient is 14 days post-abdominal surgery, and oxygen saturations are 92% on room air. The patient has not been mobilized often. Their lung sounds are clear/diminished. The patient denies cough or chest pain. You suspect this patient has:
    a. Pneumonia
    b. Pleural effusion
    c. Atelectasis
    d. Congestive Heart Failure

74. In the apneic patient, supraglottic devices can help by: [choose all that apply]
    a. Being placed without direct visualization
    b. Rapid airway intervention
    c. Providing little protection against aspiration
    d. Harming the patient if the wrong size is used

75. In the post-myocardial infarction patient, you understand that the heart wall could be damaged, causing a decrease in:
    a. Respiratory rate
    b. Hemoglobin
    c. Troponin
    d. Cardiac output

76. Your patient begins to complain of sudden onset, non-radiating, crushing chest pain that awoke him from sleep. After a focused assessment, you find no abnormalities and all vitals are normal. What is your first action?
    a. Administer loperamide, unless contraindicated
    b. Notify the cabin crew that an emergency landing is required
    c. Administer supplemental oxygen (per protocol)
    d. Dismiss the patient's complaints because your assessment was negative and vitals are stable

77. You are transporting a patient with the diagnosis of congestive heart failure (CHF) exacerbation from Chicago, Illinois, U.S. (ORD) to Mumbai, India (BOM) via Istanbul (IST). Her vitals are stable on setting 2 of the portable oxygen concentrator. Which of the following considerations are important?
    a. Patient positioning
    b. Unrestricted fluid intake
    c. Unrestricted meals
    d. Ambulating through the airports

78. You arrive at the discharging facility in Quito, Ecuador (approx. 10,000' elevation) to transport a patient with a partial small bowel obstruction. Your patient has a properly functioning naso-gastric tube in place, has positive bowel sounds, and is passing flatus and stool. The patient denies complaints. All other assessment findings are negative. Select the most appropriate statement(s) regarding the commercial transfer of this patient.
    a. The cabin altitude is less than the current altitude on the ground. The transfer is safe.
    b. The patient has bowel sounds, with a working nasogastric tube. The transfer is safe.
    c. The patient's condition is a contraindication to commercial transfer. The transfer is unsafe.
    d. The patient's bowel obstruction must be completely resolved prior to commercial transfer. The transfer is unsafe.

79. Your patient had a (L) broken hip repaired and is being repatriated home. She complains of diarrhea while traveling. Which medication is appropriate to administer?
    a. Meclizine
    b. Loperamide
    c. Ondansetron
    d. Antacid tablets

80. Your diabetic patient self-administered her insulin prior to meal service. She did not like the meal options and only ate a small amount. She is now confused and diaphoretic but can manage her airway. After measuring her blood glucose level and determining that she is hypoglycemic, which intervention is most appropriate?
    a. Encourage an additional meal
    b. Continue to monitor the blood sugar
    c. Administer oral glucose or sugary drink
    d. Declare an emergency landing

81. Your patient was SCUBA diving and upon resurfacing was confused and had slurred speech. The discharging facility performed a CT scan and the patient was diagnosed with a stroke. You understand that _____ can mimic a stroke and request a more detailed history & physical prior to transport.
    a. Arterial gas embolism
    b. Type I decompression illness
    c. Venous thromboembolism
    d. Dehydration

82. You are transporting a trauma patient with a lower extremity external fixator in place. What are some of your transport considerations? [choose all that apply]
    a. Pain management
    b. Patient positioning
    c. Easily boarding and deplaning
    d. Confirming wheelchair upon check in

83. You are transporting a 32 y/o male that has sustained 2nd degree burns to his chest and arms. He has been treated and released to a hotel by the hospital. He is fully ambulatory without assistance, vitals are stable and with the exception of the burns, his physical assessment is negative. Of the following, which is not a transport consideration?
    a. Pain management
    b. Risk of infection
    c. Mobility
    d. Nutrition & fluid balance

84. Which of the following is the most important consideration regarding drains in transport?
    a. The drain must be properly functioning
    b. The drain requires no maintenance during transport
    c. Dressings do not need to be monitored for changing
    d. Any new patient complaints are unrelated to the drain

85. Which of the following best describes a Le Forte III fracture?
    a. Transverse fracture
    b. Bridge of the nose and around the mouth
    c. Horizontal across the maxilla
    d. Orbital fracture

86. Which of the following disease processes causes a dilutional hyponatremia due to an overproduction of antidiuretic hormone from the posterior pituitary gland?
    a. Wernicke's Encephalopathy
    b. Diabetes Insipidus
    c. Central Pontine Myelinolysis
    d. SIADH

87. It is winter time and you are transporting a female patient who has cold intolerance, puffy eyelids, sparse hair, possibly goiter.   Suddenly during reassessment, she has a change in her level of consciousness. Which of the following conditions below do you suspect the patient is suffering from?
    a. Hypothyroidism
    b. Grave's Disease
    c. Cushings triad
    d. Myxedema coma

88. Which of the following answer choices is the formula to calculate MAP?
    a. ICP-SBP
    b. (2 X SBP) + DBP / 3
    c. (2 X DBP)+ SBP / 3
    d. 1/3 of the Pulse Pressure

89. A normal cerebral perfusion pressure is indicated by which of the following values?
    a. 70-90 mmHg
    b. 60-80 mmHg
    c. 60-70 mmHg
    d. 60-90 mmHg

90. Your patient presents with a blood pressure of 218/114. They deny chest pain, neurological complaints or headache. What is your impression and treatment plan? [select all that apply]
    a. This is hypertensive crisis - emergency
    b. This is hypertesive urgency - non-emergent
    c. Lower the BP more than 25% per hour
    d. Lower the BP slowly

91. Which of the following indicates left heart afterload? FMP-CDHEM-1013
    a. PVR
    b. SVR
    c. CPP
    d. PAWP

92. The cardiac output formula is defined as:
    a. Preload - Afterload
    b. SVR x CI
    c. Preload, afterload, contractile force
    d. SV x HR
    e. PCWP-DBP

93. Which of the following neurovascular statement(s) in regards to vasopressor use is incorrect? [select all that apply]
    a. α1- Vasoconstrict
    b. ß1- Dilate bronchioles & blood vessels
    c. ß2- Increase heart rate & contractility
    d. Dopaminergic – Gut kidney vessel dilation
    e. Cholinergic – Decrease heart rate

94. You arrive at the discharging facility to transport a patient that had a (R) hip repair. After your assessment, you note the patient's oral temperature to be 38 C and the chest XR to reveal lobar consolidation to the right lower lobe. Based on the information given, what is the most likely cause of the patient's condition? FMP-PULMD-1005
    a. Asthma
    b. ARDS
    c. COPD
    d. Pneumonia

95. All of the following are causes of ARDS except for which of the following?
    a. Pancreatitis
    b. Sepsis
    c. Aspiration
    d. CHF

96. You arrive at the discharging facility to transport a female patient who was recently intubated for respiratory failure and CHF exacerbation. Upon assessment, you are able to view the chest XR to confirm the correct placement of the ETT. Which of the following locations would indicate correct placement?
    a. Level of T2-T4 vertebrae
    b. Level of C7-T1 vertebrae
    c. 2-3 inches above carina on chest X-Ray
    d. 6 cm above carina on chest X-Ray

97. Which of the following is not a contraindication for the administration of Succinylcholine?
    a. History of cancer
    b. Hyperkalemia
    c. Crush Injuries
    d. Burns >24 hours

98. Which of the following medications listed below that are used in RSI have analgesic properties?
    a. Etomidate
    b. Ketamine
    c. Midazolam
    d. Propofol

99. Which of the following best describes the rapid coadministration of anesthetics and neuromuscular blockades?
    a. Rapid Sequence Induction
    b. HEAVEN
    c. Non-Invasive Positive Pressure Ventilation
    d. Delayed Sequence Intubation

100. You are transporting a 75 kg patient that is intubated and being mechanically ventilated. The patient has the following ventilator settings:

    A/C Volume
    Vt: 750 mL
    (f) 22
    Inspiratory time: 1.0 sec.
    PEEP 15 cmH2O
    FiO2 1.0

    During the flight, your high-pressure alarm begins to go off. Which of the following causes listed below could not be a cause of the high-pressure alarm?
    a. Pneumothorax
    b. Inadequate sedation
    c. Mucus plug
    d. Breath stacking
    e. Circuit disconnect

101. Select the abnormal ventilator value from the list below:
    a. VE 2-4 LPM
    b. Vt: 4-8 ml/kg/IBW
    c. FiO2 0.21-1.0
    d. PEEP 5 cmH2O
    e. pPlat <30 mmHg

102. What are the two ways to improve SPO2 in patients that are being mechanically ventilated?
    a. PEEP and FIO2
    b. Vt and (f)
    c. PEEP and (f)
    d. PS and PEEP

103. The value Pplat is a direct reflection of what?
    a. Alveolar compliance
    b. Pressure in the upper airways
    c. Acidosis
    d. VTE

104. Which of the following listed tidal volumes is within an appropriate range for a patient with an IBW of 80KG? [select all that apply]
    a. 480 ml
    b. 400 ml
    c. 320 ml
    d. 560 ml

105. You are called to transport a patient that is being mechanically ventilated. The patient is currently on the following ventilator settings:

    A/C-Volume
    Vt: 450 mL
    (f) 18
    Inspiratory time: 0.8 sec.
    FIO2 1.0
    PEEP 5 cmH2O

    While assessing the ventilator you note a Pplat of 20 and a PIP of 22. What is the next best course of action?
    a. Increase Vt
    b. Increase FIO2
    c. Decrease (f)
    d. Increase PEEP

106. This mode of ventilation gives the patient a set rate and volume. However, this mode allows the patient to draw a spontaneous breath and only take the amount of volume that the patient desires.
    a. A/C
    b. PRVC
    c. SIMV
    d. CMV
    e. APRV

ANSWER KEY

1. D
2. B
3. E
4. A, B, C
5. B
6. D
7. A, B, C, D
8. A
9. D
10. A, B, C, D, E
11. A, B, C, D
12. A
13. A
14. C
15. B, C
16. A, B, C, D
17. A, B, C, D
18. C
19. D
20. B
21. A
22. D
23. A, C
24. D
25. A
26. A
27. F
28. D
29. B
30. D
31. A
32. B, D, F
33. A
34. B
35. D
36. B
37. B
38. A, B, C,
39. B
40. C
41. G
42. A, C, D
43. A
44. A
45. A, B, C, D
46. C
47. A
48. D
49. A
50. A
51. A
52. D
53. A
54. E
55. B
56. A
57. A
58. A, B, C, D, E
59. B
60. A, B, C, D, E
61. A, C
62. A
63. A, C
64. A
65. D
66. A, B, C, D
67. A
68. C
69. A
70. A
71. A
72. C
73. C
74. A, B
75. D
76. C
77. A
78. A, B
79. B
80. C
81. A
82. A, B, D
83. C
84. A
85. A
86. D
87. D
88. C
89. A
90. B, D
91. B
92. D
93. B, C
94. D
95. D
96. A
97. A
98. B
99. A
100. E
101. A
102. A
103. A
104. A, B, C, D
105. D
106. C

REFERENCES

Aerospace Medical Association. Medical Guidlelines for Airline Travel. (2016) 3rd Edition. Retrieved from http://www.asma.org/publications/medical-publications-for-airline-travel/medical-considerations-for-airline-travel

Air & Surface Transport Nurses Association, Patient Transport Principles & Practice, Fifth Edition, . St. Louis, MO: Elsevier

American Academy of Orthopaedic Surgeons (2017) *Critical Care Transport* (2nd Ed.). Burlington, MA: Jones & Bartlett Learning

Art. 1 GDPR: Subject-matter and objectives (n.d.). Retrieved on September 17, 2020 from https://gdpr-info.eu/art-1-gdpr/

Brown, C.; Sakles, J.; & Mick, N (2018) *The Walls Manual of Emergency Airway Management* (5th Ed.). Philadelphia, PA: Wolters Kluwer

Burns, S. &, Delgado S. (2018) *AACN Essentials of Critical Care Nursing* (4th Ed.). New York, NY: McGraw-Hill

Cholera. (2019, January 17). Retrieved from https://www.who.int/news-room/fact-sheets/detail/cholera

Commission on Accreditation of Medical Transport Systems. (2019) *11th Edition Accreditation Standards*. Retrieved from https://www.camts.org/resources/

Easy in-flight exercises to prevent deep vein thrombosis. (2017, March 3). Retrieved from https://www.finavia.fi/en/newsroom/2017/easy-flight-exercises-prevent-deep-vein-thrombosis

EMTALA Fact Sheet (n.d.). Retrieved from https://www.acep.org/life-as-a-physician/ethics--legal/emtala/emtala-fact-sheet/

Farcy, D.; Chiu, W.; Marshall, J.; & Osborn, T (2017) *Critical Care Emergency Medicine* (2nd Ed.). New York, NY: McGraw Hill.

Garcia, M. (2017, September 30). How Airplane Cabin Air Works Retrieved on August 8, 2020, from https://www.travelandleisure.com/airlines-airports/how-airplane-cabin-air-works

Health Insurance Portability & Accountability Act (2019, June 13). Retrieved on September 17, 2020 from
https://www.dhcs.ca.gov/formsandpubs/laws/hipaa/Pages/1.00WhatisHIPAA.aspx

Hess, D. & Kacmarek, R. (2019) *Essentials of Mechanical Ventilation* (4th Ed.). New York, NY: McGraw-Hill.

Pagane, K. & Pagana, R. (2017) *Mosby's Manaul of Diagnostic and Laboratory Tests* (6th Ed.). St. Louis, MO: Elsevier.

Shaffner, D. & Nicholes. D. (2016) *Rogers Textbook of Pediatric Intensive Care* (5th Ed.). Philadelphia, PA: Lippincott, Williams & Wilkins.

Trotti, L. (2018, October 1) Waking up is the hardest thing I do all day: Sleep inertia and sleep drunkeness Retrieved on August 8, 2020, from
https://www.ncbi.nlm.nih.gov/pmc/articles/PMC5337178/

Weingart, S. & Borschoff, D. (2018) *The Resuscitation Crisis Manual* (1st Ed.). West Perth, W.A.: Leeuwin Press.

What is PHI? (n.d.) Retrieved on August 1, 2020 from
https://www.umassmed.edu/it/security/compliance/what-is-phi/

Photos in this book have been licensed, credited, fall under the fair use doctrine, and/or are for medical education use only

www.ingramcontent.com/pod-product-compliance
Lightning Source LLC
Chambersburg PA
CBHW051910210526
45473CB00006B/1970